PRAISE FOR
STALKED BY DEMONS, GUARDED BY ANGELS

"This memoir is honest, intelligent, and generous. I felt the heartaches and hard-won triumphs to the point where, after surfacing from an hour or two of reading, I was surprised to find I was someone else entirely. How do you make such raw, complex, personal material feel like a cozy chat over a cuppa? I'm not sure. Magic, I suspect.

"I usually read to feel entertained; Simone's book went beyond that. Reading it, I felt trusted, and that is a gift."

—**Lindsey Little**, Author of the James Munkers Series

"An inspiring and timely story told with honesty, humor, and a generous heart. Everyone knows someone—or is someone—who battles with the issues Simone explores. Here is a book to shine light on your journey."

—**Katherine Scholes**, Best-Selling Author of *The Rain Queen*

"Simone has taken a lifelong secret and transformed it into a work of art that will touch those who can relate and those who want to understand. Eating disorders are not limited to young girls; and those who struggled decades ago, without receiving the proper care, continue to struggle years later. Simone intimately shares her story and describes the strength it takes to acknowledge the eating disorder later in life. She takes an experience common to many and examines it with gentleness, honesty, and resiliency."

—**Rachael Steil**, Author of *Running in Silence: My Drive for Perfection and the Eating Disorder That Fed It*

"Well. I am on the floor. *Stalked by Demons, Guarded by Angels* is a devastating read. It was tough. I recognized so much of myself and so many women I know in the manuscript. The writing is superlative. There are so many moments of beauty and pain. It is unflinching in its gaze, and does not sugarcoat or become preachy or smugly, happily 'Look, I did it; so can you!' I started to read it and couldn't stop. I was just glued to the reading as I went and was so deeply affected by the read. It is such a work of heartbreaking beauty, with such compelling, poetic, and raw storytelling."

—**Julie Gray**, Author of *The True Adventures of Gidon Lev*

"Thank you, Simone, for your honesty. I related to your struggles and the difficulties with weight management—loving food and hating it all at the same time. Although I was not bulimic, I identified with having a dysmorphic view of myself for most if not all my life. Nothing was ever good enough, whether ten pounds lighter or heavier. I believe everyone can identify with your story. I do not know one person who does not struggle in this area. Thank you for reminding us that the answer is spiritual in nature and that we can recover a day at a time, and some days are better than others, and that is okay. Recovering from life is an inside job. The number on the scale does not matter; how big or small you are does not matter. What matters is what is in your heart. That is what makes us, not our weight. Beauty lies deep. Thank you for reminding me of that and what is important."

—**Marsha Rene**, Author of *Silencing the Enemy Within: A Memoir of Addiction and Healing*

"Simone Yemm has shared a story of frustration and pain, describing how she suffered for years from a poor self-image created by none other than the people nearest and dearest to her heart. Her story is a strong indictment of mothers that inadvertently cause their daughters pain, but also a revelation of how hope and intensive self-investigation can persevere and overcome most anything. Yemm's raw, honest, and gripping tale is worthy and especially significant to those suffering from serious eating disorders."

—**Caroline Goldberg Igra**, Author of *From Where I Stand* and *Count to a Thousand*

Stalked by Demons, Guarded by Angels;
The Girl with the Eating Disorder

by Simone Yemm

ISBN 978-1-64663-532-0

Published by

köehlerbooks™

3705 Shore Drive
Virginia Beach, VA 23455
800-435-4811
www.koehlerbooks.com

SIMONE YEMM

STALKED BY DEMONS,

GUARDED BY ANGELS

The Girl with the Eating Disorder

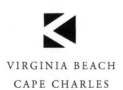

VIRGINIA BEACH
CAPE CHARLES

DEDICATION

To my familial trilogy watching from afar: June, Carrol, Vanessa

AUTHOR'S NOTE

This is my story. Told to myself, by myself. It is therefore intrinsically biased. For that, I both apologise profusely and not at all. For who should know me better than I know myself?

Time is not a linear thing and so it is with my story. Sometimes months passed like a day. Sometimes days passed like a month. As you read my story you may feel swept in and out of the present moment. This is the story of my life.

THE GENESIS

I 'm fifty-three years old. I've raised a bunch of fantastic young men and have been married twenty-seven years. I've witnessed birth. And death. Travelled in foreign countries. I have three university degrees, across two disciplines and worked for thirty-nine years in multiple capacities. I have a house, a car, and a chocolate brown Burmese cat. I'm an adult. A middle-aged woman who's lived a bit and statistically has a bit more to go.

I also have an eating disorder.

It's an incongruous label to have at my age. I'm too old for this shit. I can't speak for anyone else who struggles with any of the many varieties of eating disorders, but for me, every aspect of my existence is coloured by angst around physical appearance and my worth as a human being. I will never attain the impossible standard I set for myself.

I've been bulimic on and off since I was twenty-two, developing anorexic tendencies during a breakdown in 2016, but my war with food and body began way earlier than my twenties. I have no recollection whatsoever of having healthy eating thoughts and behaviours or positive body image and self-esteem. I'm (apparently) all grown up now, so casting blame is pointless. I'm old enough to take responsibility for my beliefs and actions. But life is rarely simple.

Developing an eating disorder is like a jigsaw puzzle—a whole gamut of pieces come together to form disordered thinking and maladaptive behaviours. This is the genesis of my personal puzzle and how I sought physical, psychological, and spiritual freedom from the chains of obsession.

IN THE BEGINNING

When I was born, I had a body.

It was white and soft and squishy, filled with all the things I need to survive. It cleverly provided the functions required to grow and develop outside the comforts of my mother's womb. What my body didn't know when it was born was that it wasn't considered the right shape or the right size. While it functioned in a beautiful, healthy, and practical manner, aesthetically it didn't conform to the ideal of beauty espoused by those who raised me and the society in which they lived.

My parents married in 1964. As is so often the case in the island state of Tasmania, they meet through mutual friends. My mother is just twenty years old, beautiful, petite, and working at LJ Hooker as a receptionist. She has a fractious and difficult relationship with her parents and is desperately seeking a way to leave behind a world of inconsistent affection, financial struggle, and her drunken, adulterous father.

My father is thirty-one years old and very close to his identical twin brother and adoring parents in Melbourne. A flautist in the Tasmanian Symphony Orchestra and professional runner, engaged twice before, passionate about music and sport, tall, dark, and handsome.

In their wedding photos, my mother has a radiant smile on her face. She's young, in love, marrying a handsome man, and making strides up her all-important social ladder. She's in the prime of youth, has a love of arts and literature, a discerning eye for beauty, a keen ear for nuance and a prodigious memory. My father is comfortable and familiar in the spotlight, with a beautiful young woman on his arm, his gentle and friendly nature loving the warm circle of affection from family and friends. Life looks complete with a successful career in music and athletics, and an adoring wife by his side. Together they seem ready to conquer the world, and the next step is to start a family.

The newlyweds buy a tiny little cottage in Jenkins Street, in the riverside suburb of Taroona. It's on a long, steep, narrow block, with a creek trickling down to the Derwent River. It's lush, green, and overgrown. Most of the land is unusable for building purposes but wild and tranquil when the newlyweds look out the sunny kitchen window in the white weatherboard cottage at the top of the block. The sounds of cockatoos, kookaburras, and the pink and grey galahs fill the little cottage with a symphony of nature's works. This is the first of many homes they will own. In this house, I'm conceived.

On Friday 25 February 1966, I'm extracted from my petite mother's womb through a high forceps delivery, weighing in at 10lb 10oz—a big, fat, healthy blob of a baby girl. This scares (and disappoints) the living daylights out of my mother. For a beautiful young woman deeply concerned about physical appearance, a fat baby (and a girl no less) is not good news. Four weeks after I am born, she tries putting a positive spin on my weight problem with her first entry in my baby book:

She has red hair, blue eyes, lashes darkening. Is beautiful now, though all her double chins are marring her beauty at present. We love her though. We will have to slim her down soon, I can see that.

And she spends the rest of her life trying to slim me down.

My father beams with pride as he drives from the Queen Alexander Maternity Hospital to the little cottage on the overgrown block, his delicate wife beside him and newborn daughter in a wicker basket on the back seat of the old Mercury Monterey. In his customary absent-minded manner, he loses his grip, drops the basket, and I roll out onto the doorstep of the sunny cottage.

Dad adores me, with my double chins and soft red hair. He's away a lot—rehearsing, performing, training, and racing—but when he's there, his face beams with pride and love. After more than half a century, I can still see it in the old black and white photos.

It's only a year before my parents and their itchy feet sell the little cottage and move across the river to build a new brick home. On Tuesday 07 February 1967, Hobart city and the surrounding areas are devastated by bushfire. While most of the fire rages on the other side of the river, even in Tranmere the embers of burnt stringybark eucalypts and Tasmanian bluegums float through the air. My mother and I are safely ensconced in the newly constructed house, sweltering through the 39°C day, while dad joins a host of other residents stamping out spot fires as they appear.

When the day is over, 2,640 square kilometres have burned, taking sixty-four lives, 62,000 livestock, innumerable native wildlife and 1,293 homes. My great grandparents lose their family home, burned to ashes on the lower slopes of Mount Wellington. But the Eastern Shore is safe and our new home unscathed in the aftermath of the Black Tuesday tragedy. For eighteen months, family life is without incident—simple and innocent with my mother planting herb gardens, making jam, and trying to tame her unruly daughter, while dad performs with the orchestra, appears on television and radio, and trains at the North Hobart Football Oval. But soon, their young family is irreparably changed.

ANGEL BABY

My baby brother has painted rosebud lips. Rouged cheeks. Long dark lashes. His face is round and perfect, crowned by wisps of dark hair. The corners of his mouth curve into a gentle smile. Five-weeks-old, with the silky soft complexion of a newborn and the double chin of a healthy, nine-pound baby. Delicate ears foreshadow a slimmer, more athletic build later in life—much like his two younger siblings to come. His eyes are softly closed, and his nose is the perfect button with a wide bridge, so familiar in an infant's face.

But it's a lie. It's all a lie.

The colours are painted onto a black-and-white photo, a common practice in the sixties. It's the only photo ever taken, in an era predating the commonality of photography we now take for granted. It was taken at the morgue sometime after he died. The soft blue background of the coloured-in photograph complements the pink cheeks and pristine white nightgown. Yet despite the false colours and two-dimensional image, it's obvious he's dead. The photograph conveys the deathly stillness of his body along with the unnatural colours of his face.

I know his story intimately well. September 17, 1968. I'm just two and a half when Christian is born at Calvary Hospital in Hobart's northern suburbs. Five weeks later, he's gone. Sudden infant death syndrome, the doctors said. A syndrome. It's not how my parents describe it. For almost three decades, we never speak of him. His photo hidden away. His death haunting my parents with grief and guilt for the rest of their days. But over the years, I learn more. Never from my mother—she rarely speaks of him and only ever in terms of how she failed. But from my father and grandmother, I piece the story together.

Christian was beautiful and healthy, chubby and full of life. His long dark lashes looked exactly like my brother, Kristin, who is yet to be conceived. Put to bed in his cot, he's later heard crying for a short period of time, but he settles himself, so my parents don't go in. For decades, they hold onto this guilt. If only . . .

When eventually dad goes in, Christian is cold and blue. No sign of the painted rosebud lips. No soft rouge on his cheeks. Just that fatal soft bluish-purple hue that skin takes on when warm blood ceases to flow through veins.

Dad shouts to my mother, "Run down to the doctor! Get the doctor now!" So she runs.

Dad desperately applies mouth-to-mouth resuscitation until the doctor arrives and tells him to stop. It's too late. He's dead. He can't be saved. The ambulance arrives and Christian is taken to the morgue. My parents don't hold him, touch him, or say goodbye. They never see him again.

My mother phones her own mother, "I've killed him! I've killed my baby!" she cries down the line.

It isn't true. But guilt is an eternal weight around every parent's neck. If only . . .

In 1968, grief counselling is a stark contrast to twenty-first-century practice. *Just have a good cry for a couple of weeks and you'll be right, dear,* say the nuns at Calvary. Buckets of tears are shed, but she is never right. My delicate mother's heart shatters into a million pieces and is never whole again.

A few weeks later, we move interstate, leaving behind all that is familiar and comforting. It's unfortunate timing. Dad has already accepted the position of Associate Principal Flautist in the West Australian Symphony Orchestra. The house is sold, packing underway, removalists organised and travel plans in place to faraway Perth. Still in the throes of grief, my parents leave friends and family behind and move 3,000 kilometres away, with me in tow, bewildered by recent events. My baby brother safely ensconced in a tiny white coffin, six feet below the earth. It's too early for the headstone to be erected before they leave, the stone masons needing more time to complete the task, but it's chosen and ordered. I know it intimately well. I've visited his grave in Hobart's Cornelian Bay a hundred times. His infant body just one in a sea of dead babies at the children's section of the picturesque riverside cemetery.

I don't remember him dying, but I have always known I had another brother. I don't remember not knowing. He's my angel brother, his round face with its gentle smile and dark lashes, never marred by age. Never naughty or disappointing. He never made mistakes or did any of the myriad things that happen as we grow and learn. He remains unchanged—forever flawless and innocent. His perfect face I've silently called upon countless times. My guardian angel with the rosebud lips and long dark lashes.

In the 1980s, my mother reads an article about cough medicine and wonders if perhaps that's how she killed her baby. She'd taken some when pregnant. For the rest of her days, she wonders what she did wrong and how things might have been different. If only . . .

In 2018, I interview my father. He's eighty-five years old and we're recording his story for posterity. Christian would have turned fifty this year. Despite five decades passing, dad cannot talk of that day without his eyes welling with tears and a catch in his throat. Still wondering how things might have been different. If only . . .

I was once asked what I would choose if I could go back in time and change one thing. Just one single thing. Without hesitation, it's this day I would change. The day my parents' hearts broke. The day my twenty-four-year-old, highly anxious mother had her worst nightmare realised. The day my emotional and sensitive father started to crack. When grief and fear began to rule our family. The day my brother became angelic and the rest of us never good enough by comparison.

FOOD RULE 01

Hide food for later.

FRIENDLY & ME

There's a castle on my wall. The bedroom ceiling is high, miles away from the top of my head. The castle has a long winding road leading up to it, surrounded by the lush, green forest of fairy tale vistas. It's a mural painted by my father and it's the most amazing work of art in the whole wide world. A fantasy world exquisitely and lovingly painted onto the bare walls of my bedroom. I love it. I go to sleep every night in a fairy tale.

By my six-year-old reckoning, I live in a huge house. The fourth since we left Tasmania in 1968. It's on stilts, typical of a 1970s Queensland home, letting cool air flow beneath the timber floorboards in the stifling Brisbane summers that are a stark contrast to the cool, temperate Tasmanian climate, 2,400 kilometres to the south. My room is long and narrow and my bed beneath the castle is close to a second door leading to my parents' bedroom. I can no longer picture their room. When I gaze back into my six-year-old self, beyond that door is black space. Beyond that door are all the lost memories of our time in Perth, where my parents desperately clung to normality and tried in vain to have another baby. And our years at Nobbys Beach on the Gold Coast, when we lived in a toy shop, I learned to read, started kindergarten and was finally presented with a new baby brother and a sister. Beyond that door are the first six years of my life—the birthday parties, temper tantrums, make-believe, and adventures I no longer recall.

I fall asleep every night talking to Friendly. Friendly is invisible and he's the bestest friend in the whole wide world. He's my only friend in the whole wide world, but I never feel alone. Friendly and I adventure into all the places I read about every day. We know all about *The Cat in the Hat*, *The Ugstabuggle*, *Winnie the Pooh*, *The Magic Faraway Tree*. We spend hours together exploring the magic and excitement of imaginary worlds, dreaming of adventures and playing with all our friends there. In these imaginary worlds, there are hugs and jelly cakes, surprises and happy endings. In these imaginary worlds, I'm always good enough.

I have a baby sister called Vanessa. She's nearly one and looks like a beautiful Japanese doll, with jet-black hair and smooth, olive skin. I have a little brother called Kristin. He's nearly two and has Vanessa's jet-black hair, but his skin is pale and freckly like mine. He has the longest dark eyelashes. Everyone comments on how exquisite his eyelashes are. Vanessa is a quiet, beautiful baby. Everyone says how beautiful she is. Kristin is hyperactive, running and climbing everywhere, never resting. Apparently, he's quite a handful. They're both so little—too young for me to play with, but I have Friendly to keep me company.

Kristin isn't the only one who's quite a handful. Mum likes everything to be just so, including her children, but our definitions of *just so* are at odds when I'm six. Familiar and comfortable in an adult world, I precociously use my extensive vocabulary to share my opinion on important matters, such as when I should go to bed and how much food I'll eat. I'm labelled headstrong, determined, stubborn, inquisitive, active—not in the least bit fearful to set out anywhere and anytime I please, to adventure with Friendly into the lands of make-believe.

Dad, with his rose-coloured glasses, remembers me as a good child, always a doer and a leader, never a follower. But mum is concerned with my level of wilful stubbornness and takes me to a psychologist who declares me perfectly normal, though quiet and withdrawn, and proclaims, "She'll look after you." And I learn to look after everyone.

Vanessa and Kristin look so similar, almost like twins. I look nothing like them. My skin is fair and freckly and I'm chubby. I've always been chubby. Everyone says so. But grandma says it's puppy fat that will mysteriously disappear when I get older. I can't wait to get older. My hair is a mess of thick, red curls mum always tries to straighten. Grandma loves my curls though, and teaches me a rhyme,

There was a little girl, who had a little curl,
Right in the middle of her forehead.
When she was good, she was very, very good,
But when she was bad, she was horrid.

I spend lots of time with grandma now that Vanessa and Kristin are born. She teaches me to read, and she loves animals and gardens. She always has biscuits and lollies at her house. Friendly and I dip our hands into the jars when she's not looking and hide them away for a secret party later on. Sometimes I stay with her for weeks and weeks when I've become too much of a handful. She doesn't live with Grandpa Maurice anymore. I don't know why. Nobody talks about him. I don't remember him.

On my chubby six-year-old legs, I walk two blocks to the corner shop. It seems a long way but I'm happy to be entrusted to walk all by myself to bring back a long-forgotten *very important item*. I love being alone, free to wander without care or supervision. I've always loved wandering and adventuring, long before I can remember.

Family lore says the milkman brought me home when I was three, after I let myself out the front door and wandered off to explore the neighbourhood, my parents still snug in their bed, asleep. At five, Friendly and I packed all my white socks into a little red tin lunch box and ran away from home—until we got hungry and came back. A year later, I caught the wrong bus home from school, realised my mistake, then followed my nose and set off, walking two suburbs across Brisbane to get home, just as the police came looking for me. I had no idea what all the fuss was about. I saw a problem and came up with a perfectly reasonable solution. In all my years, I've never been afraid to pack up, set off, and see what happens. What happens has not always been what I expected.

RASPBERRY JUBES

Friendly and I are in our land of daydreams, walking to the old white weatherboard house, converted into a corner store with a bit of everything essential—milk in glass jars, bread in paper bags, newspapers stacked high. And my favourite thing, Jaffas that cost just one cent for three. The shopkeeper knows me. It isn't the first time I've been sent on a *very important errand*, and she smiles as I leave with my Jaffas. I finish them one after the other, crunching through the hard orange candy and sucking up the smooth soft chocolate on the inside.

Friendly and I count silently as we walk, turning everything into multiples of three, because three is a very important number. We count the steps between cracks in the pavement, always in threes. We rearrange the spelling of words so the letters are in threes. We collect gumnuts and frangipanis in groups of three. Numbers are important but I don't know why.

As I head back down the cool leafy street, a man walks up alongside me. He looks like a giant, at least eight feet tall with short dark hair and a long dark coat.

"Hello, little one. What pretty hair you have!"

People always like my hair with its soft Shirley Temple curls, carroty red in the afternoon winter sun. Except my mother. She still brushes it into unwieldy pigtails every chance she gets.

"Would you like a lolly?"

He holds out a brown paper bag. Oh my. Of course, I want a lolly! My hand is twitching, desperate for a lolly, the sugary delight of the Jaffas still fragrant in my mouth.

"Go on. You can have as many as you want."

I want them all and I can almost taste them on my lips. Raspberry jubes peak out of the bag—the heady scent of sugary heaven wafting my way. I want those lollies.

I walk down the street with Friendly invisibly and silently by my side, the giant man walking with us. We don't know what to say. I want those lollies, but what if he poisoned them? My six-year-old head is busy processing every possibility of this unexpected scenario. *Don't talk to strangers. Don't be rude. Ignoring people is rude. But what if he poisoned the lollies?* I ask Friendly what to do but he doesn't know, so I don't say anything at all. We keep on walking while the man is chatting away.

"Are you sure you don't want some?" he insists.

A dark blue sedan pulls up next to us and the driver winds her window down. I have no idea who the lady is, but she looks old. Even older than my mother.

"Are you okay, Simone? Do you want a lift home?"

She knows my name. I don't know how she knows my name. I would never get in a car with a stranger. Friendly and I keep walking, but the man has walked away now. He took the lollies with the raspberry jubes, and he went the other way.

"No, thank you. I'm almost home."

The lady in the blue car watches me cross the road and walk up the steep path overgrown with kangaroo grass, fruit trees, and flowering gums to our front door. I'm not sure if I'm relieved or disappointed. I like being with grownups but it's weird for strangers to talk to me. I really did want those lollies. There are no lollies at our house—ever. We only eat healthy vegetarian food like lentils and spinach. I take the *very important item* back to my mother cooking in the big sunny kitchen and the rest of the day passes in a blur.

"Simone!"

It's nine o'clock at night. I'm never allowed up this late.

"Wake up. We need you to talk to the policeman. Tell him about the man who talked to you when you went to the shop."

The man? Have I done something wrong? I've never had a policeman visit me before. I feel like a grownup. He talks to me for ages, asking what the man looked like and where he came from and where he went and what did he say. But I'm not in trouble. The lady in the blue car rang my parents and they rang the police. A suspicious man in a dark coat has been looking for small children lately. I guess those lollies were probably poisoned.

DANCE TO THE SILENT BEAT

I t's 1975, almost a year since we arrived back from a brief sojourn to the Canary Islands—memories of gypsies, cave houses, near-drownings, and evenings in a Spanish bar watching dad perform with the local musicians still fresh in my mind. We're back in the Apple Isle living in house number nine—one house for each of my nine years.

Before buying our new home in Howrah, we spend six months living in the tiny beachside community of South Arm where I'm introduced to music for the first time. Dad loans me his precious silver Haynes piccolo, small enough for my fingers to manage, and teaches me to play. Friendly and I disappear together for hours on end to discover the excitement of learning to make music.

In a letter to my grandmother, he writes:

Simone loves the small school she goes to. In the three weeks she has been playing the piccolo, we have not had to force her to practice & she is very promising. Simone does at least one hour practice a day (1/2 hour before school & 1/2 hour after). I just spend a few minutes each time with her & she is happy to keep going. Her repertoire consists of five scales & arpeggios, several small tunes including "God save the queen" & "O come all ye faithful," also a duet which we play together. You would be proud of your granddaughter. She may be able to sit alongside me as 2nd flute & piccolo one day.

I meet Kerry in grade five at Howrah Primary School. As we've traversed thousands of miles and moved state several times, I've somehow ended up in a class with students one to two years older than me. Kerry lives a short walk from our house, and we soon become firm friends, a friendship that continues to this day. Her family is so different from mine. She's the youngest of three and I'm envious of her youngest child status that comes with more freedom and fewer responsibilities. Her mum is always cooking and gardening, making preserves and sewing dresses.

At their house, there are sausages and mashed potatoes, sponge cakes and white bread. Food is in abundance and always on offer. Our house is filled with lentils and spinach and fresh fruit—loads of apricots, greengages, apples, and raspberries on display, but consumption requires hard-earned permission. My mother is a wonderful cook, turning dull looking lentils into delicious soups served with wholegrain breads and real butter.

Suburban Howrah is built on the remnants of old apricot orchards and the houses have ancient apricot trees that produce fat, dark, sweet, juicy fruit that's soon turned into jam, preserves, and apricot crumble. Kerry and I start our first business, with a handmade sign and a set of scales from my other grandmother, setting up shop on the footpath selling bags of apricots. We make $7 each in the first two days—good money for not much effort in 1975. When we're not selling our parents' hard-grown fruits or handmade lavender bags, Kerry and I play with Barbie dolls at her house, swim in the brisk Derwent River, walk her dogs, share our Holly Hobby swap cards, and roam the neighbourhood riding bicycles and collecting banana passionfruit. I finally have a friend—a real friend— and it isn't long before I completely forget how Friendly looks and sounds.

I'm no longer satisfied with the classical and jazz music dad performs and my mother prefers. Like most kids, I want to listen to the music of my generation and ABBA are at the top of my list. Along with The Bay City Rollers, Meatloaf, and Racey. Annafried and Agnetha are the very picture of perfection with their body-hugging white outfits and styled poofy hair. I save my pocket money, purchase LPs and memorise every single word.

Details of my parents' sojourns have long since lapsed from memory, but their absence one evening is a picture-perfect recollection. They walk out the door, dad handsome and respectable in his suit and tie. My tiny mother dolled up in the height of 1970s fashion with her flared, high-waisted trousers. Vanessa and Kristin are just four and five, and as usual, run amok for the babysitter.

I head to my bedroom at the end of the hallway and close the door. There's a giant built-in wardrobe on the left connected to my brother's bedroom, like a trip through the forest of Narnia coats I've read about again and again. My white wooden bed is flush against the wall and standing tall in the middle of the room is a free-standing full-length swivel mirror. I haven't yet learned to avoid my reflection, and instead, find myself standing in front of the mirror, gazing into the future with the freedom to be whomever I please, and do whatever I want. Today I'm a dancer. Despite my puppy fat, dearth of dancing lessons and complete absence of ability, I have faith in the endless possibility of dreams coming true.

My head reverberates with silent music. Perhaps it was Tchaikovsky's *Swan Lake*, Andrew Lloyd Webber's *Jesus Christ Superstar* or ABBA's *Mamma Mia*. But I like to think it was *I do, I do, I do*.

My young body moves and sways, twists and twirls with deep contentment. I'm a dancer. On stage. On my own. Encased in warm light and surrounded by infinite darkness. There's an invisible audience beyond the edge of the stage. They watch without judgment, a young girl expressing the depths of her soul through every inch of her body. My hair twirls, hips sway, and feet spin with ease and freedom. I'm happy. I'm alone in my room, encased in a cocoon of hope, dreams, and endless possibilities. I can be anyone I want, and at this moment in time, I choose to stand in the spotlight on stage, expressing every suppressed emotion through the movement of my body. I'm in love with the reflection of movement and freedom.

I dance to the silent beat until exhaustion overcomes me and I collapse into bed for the night, dreaming dreams of the dancer's life.

Breakfast is always an early affair. Three hyperactive children rarely sleep late, and my parents are early risers. Dad's at work as usual, my mother pottering in the kitchen while the three of us sit at the bench with its iconic seventies burnt orange laminate and brown wooden cupboards. My mother prepares a simple breakfast of cereal, toast, home-made marmalade, stewed nectarines and home-made yoghurt. And orange juice. Always orange juice. She looks at me and starts to laugh.

"We saw you last night."

I have no idea what she's talking about.

"We were parked in the driveway watching you stare at yourself in the mirror. You looked like you were having fun. Were you pretending to be a dancer?"

My heart thumps so hard, I think it will burst from my chest. My pulse doubles, body freezes, and brain ceases to function. I say nothing.

"Did you realise you'd left the curtains open? Anybody could have seen you."

Fight, flight, freeze—the body's natural response to danger. My body always freezes, including my tongue. I don't know what to say, but I feel a flush of shame deep in my belly, rising to colour my cheeks magenta. I shovel my Weet-Bix in even faster.

Thoughts race at my stupidity. My naivete for believing I was safe and alone in my bedroom. My private delusions of grandeur on public display, and to my mother of all people. She busies herself with the rest of breakfast and her immaculate cleaning of the kitchen, oblivious to the massive internal shift in my belly. Time after time, my dreams and emotions are shattered and mocked. I feel a little snap in my head.

I never trust her again.

FOOD RULE 02

Steal food when no-one's looking.

BODY OF SHAME

Mutual trust and respect disappear, if indeed they ever existed, between me and my mother. Despite my wilfulness and persistency, she holds all the power. After all, she's thirty-one and I'm nine. I miss Friendly and having someone to talk to about anything. He disappeared like Casper the Ghost, soon after we left South Arm, right around the time I met Kerry.

Another conflict arises, the details of which have long since passed from memory, and for the first time, I wish I'm dead. I'm wearing my favourite denim pinafore, standing in our living room with its full-length windows looking out over my mother's manicured vegetable and herb gardens, and the giant old apricot and walnut trees. I don't want to run away—it never works out and I always come back. This time, I want to be dead, but I don't know how. She buried one child long ago and while it's never discussed, I'm acutely aware of how painful that loss was. My death seems a fitting way to punish her for the long-forgotten conflict between us, and an apt way to remove myself from a family in which I don't belong. It's another decade before I'm knowledgeable enough to make an attempt, but the thought plants a dark seed, and when life feels unbearable, it becomes an automatic thought pattern—*I wish I was dead*.

The inside of my head is a noisy place. It always has been. Years spent buried in books filled with characters and adventures, dreams and disasters, fantasy and folly, leave me with a head full of wishes and wilfulness and the enduring capacity to visualise every tasty morsel I soak up from the weathered paperback novels.

Some days, I dream of my life as a dancer, singer, famous author, or—most commonly—a professional flautist just like my dad. The feeling's almost tangible, with a sense of comfort and inevitability nestled deep inside my chest. A secret I share with nobody for fear of mocking.

Other days, my inner world is a catastrophe. I'm too stupid, too fat, too shy, ugly, clumsy, unworthy. I'll never deserve or achieve a dream and the vividly imagined reality of shame, humiliation, and the desperate search for love and acceptance burrows into the secret nest of emotions in my chest. Unshed salty tears silently spill on my death wish, feeding a desire to be at peace. To feel nothing. And always, always wondering, *Will anybody care if I'm gone?*

A new house is built behind ours and a family with two young girls move in. They're labelled troublemakers by my mother, and I'm discouraged from playing with them. Her opinion makes them all the more appealing, and we spend even more time together over the next three years. I'm desperate to please my mother and be praised for being good, while steadfastly refusing to bend to her will. When she grabs a wooden spoon to smack my backside for a misdemeanour, I snatch it out of her hand and hit her back. It's the last time she ever hits me. I'm twelve years old.

Before I know it, the girls next door teach me to shoplift. I start by inadvertently seeing sleight of hand at the newsagent and handfuls of lollies appearing for our delightful consumption soon after. There's a deep knowing in my gut that it's very, very wrong but I have friends now and friends are more important. I witness a few more incidents before I'm dared to steal something for them in return—fair is fair, apparently. I nervously mimic the sleight of hand witnessed at the newsagency and triumphantly share the stolen musk sticks and Twisties with the girls, while secretly ashamed of the way I have treated the innocent newsagent. They were not mine to take. My mother was right all along; those girls were troublemakers. I refuse to acknowledge her wisdom.

Easter rolls around and I spontaneously decide to steal an Easter egg as a gift for my mother. I wander into the department store on my own and nervously stroll the aisles for what seems like hours, vacillating between the sense of wrongness and the joy I can picture on my mother's face when I gift her the egg. I gather a little courage, hide the egg in my schoolbag, and head to the exit.

I'm caught. The police are called, and my life of crime comes to an abrupt end. Dad arrives at the police station to collect me—a rare look of anger on his face when we pull into the driveway. It's the first and last time I remember being smacked by him and I disappear to my room in tears of shame, the sting of his anger worse than his hand. My mother comes in with a rare look of sympathy on her face and puts her arm around me. It's the first and last time I remember being comforted by her. My body freezes, heart races, and cheeks flush crimson. Concrete evidence of my failure to be good—to be perfect, as my grandmother always reminds me. My mother's arm around me feels so foreign, I can't bear it. I hold still until she leaves, then crawl into bed and cry myself to sleep. I never shoplift again.

The girl next door laughs at my failure, then randomly asks, "How much do you weigh?"

I hesitate, knowing I'm fat and unpleasant to look at, so she tells me she's eight stone. There's a little spark of elation in my chest as I realise we're the same weight—perhaps I'm not fat and ugly?! She bursts out laughing at my gullibility and confesses she's only six stone. Her tiny petite frame beneath a head of snow-white curls not obvious to me until the humiliation of the sharing.

In the 1960s, thin was in. Twiggy was the new kid on the runway, and slim, athletic builds were admired and to be attained. As I grow, my voluptuous curves never stand a chance. I'm not thin enough or pretty enough. My skin is too fair, my hair too red. I grow too tall, too round, and my breasts too large. I don't know all this when I'm born, but I don't remember not knowing. It's the story I hear since the day I first draw breath.

Weight is a topic that's always on the table. I have too much of it. I eat too much. I'm too lazy. I crave the wrong foods. I live in a family of beautiful people, and I have beautiful tiny friends. Beauty is the essential ingredient on the path to success in life, and as my body size is unacceptable, so is every aspect of my appearance. I start wallowing in self-pity about the fact that I'll never be thin or pretty—my internal catastrophising fanning the death wish flames.

As I grow from child to teen, I add more angst and humiliations to the list. I go to the toilet frequently. As a fifty-year-old, I learn urinary frequency and urgency have a name—overactive bladder syndrome. As a child, I learn it's because I'm too lazy to wait. Trips to the bathroom are monitored, and my inability to wait is met with disappointment on good days and anger on bad days. I associate going to the bathroom with embarrassment and shame and avoid going if anyone is around, leading to more urgency and accidents. The onset of menstruation and the long, heavy, painful periods I experience for twenty-five years add to the horror of my uncontrolled, unruly, unlovable body.

Humiliation becomes as commonplace as my self-pity, but neither deter my wilful desire to do as I please, too stubborn to let even my sense of self-worth come between me and the things I want to do.

FOOD RULE 03

If I see it, I must eat it.

JEKYLL & HYDE

In 1978, I move to my sixth educational institution, commencing grade seven at Hobart's Ogilvie High School—an all-girls' school my mother attended twenty years earlier. IQ tests are standard practice for grade six students in the 1970s and high schools are streamed. I'm placed into 7A, because despite my lacklustre interest in study, apparently I'm smart enough to be there. My reports remain lacklustre throughout high school.

My friendship with Kerry is strong and enduring, while the girls next door—much to my mother's relief—drift away as we move to different schools. My friendship circle is small, but life is busy and full. Flute playing is an integral part of my routine, and I find a community of adults and peers who share a common interest. I perform in eisteddfods, play in bands and orchestras, and attend flute society activities and events. I fit in. I win prizes, pass exams, and make dad proud. Music is an integral part of my identity, and I revel in every moment spent with dad and away from my mother's judgment—soaking up all the knowledge he imparts to his students, unknowingly immersed in a first-class teaching apprenticeship.

I'm part of a small friendship group at the start of grade seven. My two years at Ogilvie are filled with all the normalities of blossoming into a teenager—angst over the appearance of breasts, pubic hair, and menstrual periods (all mortifying events); anxiety around friendships and how I fit in; ongoing conflict with my mother over how to dress, speak, eat, sleep, look, behave, exist; a budding awareness of the vagaries of the male species, but in an all-girls' school, no opportunity to learn boys are, in fact, not as peculiar as they may at first seem. There's no repeat of my shoplifting antics, but I remain easily led astray, desperate to fit in and belong. I smoke cigarettes at lunchtime. We practice hyperventilating until we pass out. A small group of us decide to spray Pure & Simple, a household cooking spray, into plastic bags, then inhale the contents. The school principal finds out and individually calls us to his office where we're shown a chemistry set and invited to drink random poisons. When we look shocked, he asks how it's any different. I never sniff Pure & Simple— or any other noxious chemicals—again.

Music is central to my world, inside and outside school, but away from music, I'm isolated and alone. I'm not pretty, slim, or fashionable. I yearn to be as slim and pretty as my friends, so I naively attempt to dress like them—despite clearly having a different body shape and colouring. I dress for their body types, emphasising my lumps and bumps, bringing a deep sense of shame at my ugliness. Vanessa is an adorable seven-year-old, praised for her natural-born beauty. A curtain of glossy black hair crowns her perfect face. I've learned to straighten my hair, styling it into truly appalling Farah Fawcett flicks, while I spend evenings putting my little sister's hair in rags to create a cascade of beautiful curls. We both learn that whatever we're blessed with, it isn't enough.

By the time I'm officially a teenager, my relationship with food is much like my relationship with my mother—utterly dysfunctional. I can't pass a morsel of food without a compulsion to eat it. My great aunt is mystified when I hide Iced VoVo biscuits under the pillow at her house. My mother is appalled when she catches me eating food off the ground. Nobody knows I take second, third, or fourth helpings and disappear to the toilet, eating in desperation and shame. All my pocket money is spent on food. To avoid being seen eating, I hide in public toilets and consume my treasures, carefully disposing of wrappers silently and invisibly so nobody knows.

Music features in my daily routine but sports do not. I'm very active walking and bicycling, my energy levels sky-high, but I'm not considered sporty, and a blooming bosom does nothing to encourage me to run. As children, I'm deemed musical while my siblings are athletic. It takes decades before it dawns on me that my father is both a professional musician and a professional athlete; one does not preclude the other. Still, the seed is sown. I'm distinctly fearful of sporting activities—a fear that my weight, bouncing boobs, and presumed non-athleticness will make me an object of humiliation.

At various times, my mother and grandmother pull me aside to chat about my weight problem. I look at photos of my thirteen-year-old self and see a girl with terrible fashion sense, a bad haircut, and an awful lot of freckles. A body with a solid build filling out into an hourglass shape, very different from the rest of my slim family who bypassed the puppy fat phase. But I was never grotesquely overweight. My weight problem was morphing into a food obsession, driven by a compulsion to numb emotions threatening to expose me as vulnerable.

My mother and grandmother focus on modifying my eating behaviours—encouraging me to eat less. Less food, less often, less delicious—in the hope there would be less of me. I'm being primed for an eating disorder, and it's simply a matter of which path I take—restriction, starvation, over-exercising, and anorexia? Or binging, overeating, purging, and bulimia? I'm too rebellious to acquiesce to my mother's desires, and my boobs are too big to comfortably exercise, so I eat every chance I can—to spite her. And I hate myself for it.

My entrance into the teenage years is a Jekyll and Hyde experience— my outer world full, busy, confident, and competent and my inner world consumed with doubt, angst, self-loathing, and worthlessness. I don't know who I am.

GRUBBY PRINCE

In 1980, millions of viewers around the world are wondering, *Who Shot J R?* while I'm the new kid in year nine at Ballina High School on the beach-laden New South Wales north coast. Dad is now a full-time lecturer at the University in Lismore, and his days of regular absences from the family home come to an end. We're a long way from Tasmania's four-seasons-in-a-day climate and most of my cable knits and woollen vests are soon replaced with boob tubes and short shorts. I'm still dressing my curvy body in skinny-girls' fashion.

I farewell Tassie friends as we pack up and move 3,000 kilometres away. There are promises we'll always write and never lose touch. Social media and mobile phones are decades away from everyday usage, so staying in touch requires interstate phone calls (expensive and I'm not allowed to make them) or putting pen to paper and posting it off. Most of my friends eventually move on and disappear into the vagaries of distant memory. My friendship with Kerry endures.

I swan into adolescence, still waiting for the puppy fat to disappear as grandma promised. My mother is increasingly frustrated with my undignified body and offers incentives to lose weight. Before leaving Tasmania, she's promised me $5 for every pound I lose—a veritable fortune for a thirteen-year-old in late 1979—but first I have to lose five pounds. I don't lose a single ounce.

A year later, I'm sent to Weight Watchers where I again fail to lose an ounce of fat, but now I have to sit in the piggy corner as evidence of my failure. I'm the only teenager in the back room of a community hall, full of middle-aged overweight women and one leader. I remember not one single word ever spoken, or any useful advice. The meal plans are somewhat obsolete for a teenager, as I do none of the cooking at home. And the list of do-nots far outweigh any sense of joy. Whatever the premise of the programme in the 1980s, it makes no impact on my eating awareness and certainly never mentions a connection between emotions and food. I'm not always alone in the piggy corner; sometimes I'm joined by equally embarrassed women twice my age.

Enroute to Ballina, I stay with my aunt and uncle in Melbourne for a short while. I'm utterly mortified to wake one morning and discover my period has arrived and there are stains on the sheets. Just a few spots, but there's no hiding it, so I take a deep breath to quell the tears and shaking hands, then traipse downstairs to share this humiliating piece of information with my aunt. She has a quick look, wonders what all the fuss is about, helps me change the bed, and asks if I need any pads. I love her even more for gifting me a momentary sense of acceptance and normality.

I adore our house in Ballina—number eleven since I first rolled onto the doorstep at Jenkins Street in Taroona. It's not the rendered whitewashed walls or the banana trees and custard apples growing in the tropical rainforest of our suburban garden that I love, it's the fact I have not just a bedroom, but a whole flat to myself.

Upstairs is a three-bedroom home, paying tribute to the '70s with orange and yellow shagpile carpet my mother hates and lacquered kitchen cork tiles I accidentally set fire to a couple of years later. Downstairs is my haven for four whole years—an unprecedented period of time in one location for our family. Accessed through the converted garage with sliding glass doors protecting the huge blue ping-pong table, the door at the back leads to my bedroom, freshly painted in lemon yellow. It's big— way bigger than average—and soon papered with my poetry and posters of poofy-haired teen celebrities torn from Dolly magazines.

I have a lounge room next door where my flute and piano are housed, and a Space Invaders machine is later ensconced. I can play ninety-nine games for free, then lift the glass lid and reset for another ninety-nine games. The hours spent mastering the art of shooting down pixelated spacecraft is a testament to my single-minded, obsessive pursuit of (pointless) perfection.

The kitchen, painted the same lemon yellow but flooded with daylight from the white timber windows, opens onto stairs leading to the outdoor bathroom and family laundry, fragrant with the scent of frangipanis in the garden. A full bladder at 2 a.m. is an inconvenient trek, but otherwise, I love my space. And it's all mine—much to my siblings' disgust.

Ballina High School is huge. There are over 1,000 students from grades seven-twelve and approximately half of them are boys—a completely foreign species to me. Most students have been there since grade seven and friendship groups are well established. Nevertheless, I find a group of girls willing to accept me and I soon slip into the everyday humdrum of high school life. My musical and writing abilities are more advanced than most of my peers and I find comfort in music and English classes. The rest of my curriculum is uninteresting, and I put in no effort whatsoever, disappointing my parents and teachers.

For the first time, I perform in school musicals and fall in love with the theatre. Costumes, hairdos, stage makeup, and false eyelashes, lights, microphones, cameras, and curtains. The fantasy worlds of make-believe explored in hundreds of my books are brought to life in vivid colour. I'm not a star performer—performance and social anxiety induce too much self-doubt to ever do well in auditions. But I'm deliriously happy in the chorus, small groups, and the occasional small part here and there. I'm also happy in the band, and beyond thrilled when I have the opportunity two years later to perform next to my father for the first time—second flute in the band for the Lismore production of Don Quixote.

Before the year is out, dad accrues too many flute students and deems me advanced enough to take on a few beginners. I'm thirteen when I commence teaching. My first students don't benefit from great wisdom or teaching techniques, but with my father's unintentional apprenticeship, and his endless patience to answer questions and assist me as required, I eventually grow into a respected teacher and develop an enormous love of mentoring and teaching young people.

At fifteen, I have a blossoming libido (that blossom has since bloomed, withered, and died). Still an avid reader, I dream of finding my prince. Not literally. I think I'd fall off my non-literal horse if a prince came my way. But if a cute (or non-cute) guy looked at me twice, I would be the luckiest gal on the planet. There's just one problem—I'm too self-absorbed with revulsion at my red hair, fair skin, double D breasts, and size fourteen thighs to notice any noticing.

My first encounters with boys are fleeting and unpleasant—a random guy shoving his hand up my skirt and grabbing my crotch at a Midnight Oil performance in the Ballina RSL Club. My friend's older cousin pushing his fat fingers inside my knickers after getting us drunk on cheap port. Then my first dalliance. And it's most certainly not with a prince.

My pale white ass sits on the cracked, green vinyl backseat of an old bus from Ballina to Lismore, with its week-old chewing gum stuck to the sweaty seats and *T loves C* in permanent marker on the bench seat in front of me. As passengers disembark, the subtropical rainforest bends recede into the background and the familiar flood-prone township of Lismore starts to appear in front. A teenage boy—whose name I'll thankfully never know—sidles closer, as does his wandering hand, which finds its way beneath my much-too-short, pale blue uniform and worms its grubby little way towards my knickers. He's feeling me up. I'd never thought it could happen to me.

Not a word is spoken. No introductions. No smiles across a candlelit dinner. My first dalliance with a boy is being touched up on the backseat of a public bus. Eventually, he's brazen enough to kiss me. My first kiss— discarded with as much care as a used tissue. Tossed into the nearest rubbish bin, full of bad smells and bad memories. His wandering hands multiplying rapidly and everywhere at once—thighs and breasts, belly and chin. Firm pressure. Squeezing for his pleasure and exploration.

And always with his mouth pressed onto mine—stale teenage boy breath exhaling into my lungs.

I'm deeply self-conscious and consumed with mixed emotions.

Finally, a boy has noticed me, while the bus driver watches in the mirror. *What does he expect from me? What happens next? I don't know what to do. I have my period! How can I tell him? I don't know what to do.*

I'm uncomfortable in this situation, and it's almost time to get off the bus. I don't know what to do.

As those grubby fingers—a literal phrase, his nails completely embedded with dirt—slowly make their way beneath my yellow daisy knickers, I see the bus driver eyeing us in his mirror, and the last turns through the streets of Lismore are upon us.

I dig deep—very deep—into my pitiful pool of courage and speak the only six words I recall either of us sharing, "I'm sorry. I have my period."

We pull apart. Straighten our clothes as though nothing happened. Say nothing and don't look at each other again. I exit the old green bus and mumble a *thank you* to the driver.

I'm struck dumb with shame—shame at my body for being grotesque and bleeding at inappropriate moments, for being so abhorrent it's only desirable to smelly vagrant teenagers on the backseat of a bus, shame at myself for being touched in such a public place and manner and being too weak to say no, shame at knowing the bus driver saw the whole episode—*Does he know who I am? Does he know my dad?*—shame at my body for responding in such a manner, being simultaneously aroused and revolted, shame at the very core of my being—and a tiny, tiny little spark inside me that says, *a boy noticed me.*

GROWING UP

My relationships with boys are sad and sorry but my friendships start to mature. Kerry and I still write, and despite the vast distance and prohibitive travel costs, she flies from Hobart to Ballina to visit.

Like most of the close bonds I eventually form in life, no amount of time or distance changes our friendship; when she steps off the plane, we pick up right where we left off. Except the Holly Hobby swap cards are swapped for body surfing in the big surf and comparing notes on our favourite popstars. Kerry is a girl like me in so many ways—tall and curvy with boobs and hips. But she's also beautiful, a fact my mother cannot help but notice. I no longer recall the conversations or observations from my mother, but thirty-five years later, Kerry remembers how mortified she felt when I was compared unfavourably to her slimmer, fitter figure, fearing I'd hate her for the comparison and no longer want to be friends. Despite her best efforts, my mother has never been able to have much input in my friendships.

In a world predating instant messaging and mobile phones, I'm alone and safe with my thoughts when Kerry goes home. I practise the flute and piano, or curl up in bed for hours on end, reading anything I get my hands on to escape the fears running out of control in my hormonal teenage head. I rehash early childhood favourites like *The Secret Garden* and *The*

Magic Pudding or escape into my newfound love of fantasy in *Lord of the Rings* or the titillating naughtiness of *Puberty Blues*.

I finish my high school years in this house, safe in my little cocoon downstairs while life upstairs spirals out of control. Vanessa transitions from an adorable eight-year-old at the start of 1980 to an out-of-control, mentally unstable twelve-year-old when I leave in December 1983, her beauty no protection against the dysfunctional relationships within our family. My parents, desperate to maintain control of her increasingly erratic behaviour, are battered and broken. Their much-longed-for relocation to sunshine, surf beaches, and serenity inadvertently shatters our family apart as they struggle to navigate the distress of raising an out-of-control child with no external support.

Kristin loses his close bond with Vanessa and becomes immersed in a world of easy friendships. He's a good student and a lovable personality. He's popular, sporty, smart, and mostly ignored at home. Caught between an older sister escaping into a world of music and teaching, and a younger sister no longer capable of functioning in civilised society, he's left to his own devices to grow into his teenage years.

For all intents and purposes to the outside world, our house is home to an average middle-class family of five. But behind the painted white doors, we're a family torn apart by unrecognised mental health issues, at a time when it's easier to win at Space Invaders than to access psychological support.

In December 1983, I pack all my precious possessions into our beige Volkswagen Passat and drive to Brisbane in search of new adventures, vowing and declaring I will never—under any circumstance—move back to that house. I'm true to my word.

I arrive in Brisbane with my closest high school friend, where we set ourselves up in a tiny flat, find a job selling house cladding door-to-door, and revel in the heady delights of living without parental supervision.

After a few exhausting weeks of traipsing the streets, being bitten by a dog, collapsing in the heat, and earning precisely zero dollars, a taxi driver pulls over and asks if I want a lift home. I clarify my financial situation and say I'm happy walking, but he kindly tells me it isn't a problem and will drop me home anyway. In my naivete, I consider it an act of gentlemanly charity. When we get to my flat, he insists I kiss him goodbye to thank him for his generosity. I'm once again caught in an uncomfortable situation where I know it's wrong, can't deal with conflict, don't want to be rude, and have no idea how to extricate myself. I kiss the creepy middle-aged taxi driver, my second kiss disposed of with as much care and passion as the first. I quit my career as a door-to-door salesperson.

I visit a local doctor for reasons I no longer recall, and while there, he convinces me I need a pap smear and breast examination. I've never had either before and haven't been seen naked by another human being since I was a little girl being bathed by grandma. I'm instructed to strip naked and lie uncovered on the examination table where the little old Jewish doctor somehow manages to perform both procedures simultaneously. My face flushes and I stare at the floor as I exit the surgery. It's a great many years before I'm brave enough to have either examination done, and never again by a man. My dream of finding a knight in shining armour is evaporating as I decide my unacceptable body makes me unworthy of normal relationships; I'm somehow tainted and only suitable for creepy dudes in buses, taxis, and doctor examination tables.

My obsession with the number three has stayed with me since childhood, but I've added new methods of keeping the inside of my head quiet and busy. Long before I learn of Mr. Fibonacci and his famous mathematical sequence, I practise his numbers. When shame and disgust descend upon me, I start adding number upon number—anything to escape the emotions I cannot bear. Memories of boys and old men are fast replaced with ever-increasing Fibonacci numbers. It seems being an adult is filled with as many unpleasantries as all my other life stages to date.

Despite our measly budget, we still find the means to socialise, and one weekend, we make the one-hour drive from Brisbane to the tourist-laden Gold Coast and its infamous sand, surf, and sunshine. We have a few drinks, hit the nightclubs, and before we know it, pick up a couple of guys. We spend the rest of the night with them in the club, watch the sunrise over Surfers Paradise beach wrapped in strong tanned arms, then drive back to Brisbane with our new friends.

My housemate and her beau soon disappear, while the gorgeous surfer dude squeezes into a little single bed with me. Finally, an encounter with a boy that doesn't make me feel dirty—exciting, joyous, full of lovely soft kisses and holding hands on the beach—but I'm naive, inexperienced, and have no idea how to handle myself. I'm too afraid to do anything, so wait for things to happen. Surfer dude, and his sun-bleached curls, is too gentlemanly to be presumptuous, so we spend the night curled up together hugging, kissing, and falling asleep at uncomfortable angles. I'm astonished at the turn of events, embarrassed by my lack of worldliness, and disappointed nothing else happened. My golden opportunity missed because I'm too afraid to say what I want or ask what to do. And he was too polite to say what he wanted and tell me what to do. But a little chink of optimism cracks through my protective armour of ugliness—that perhaps one day I'll find a nice guy.

FOOD RULE 05

Eat so fast that nobody notices.

ANXIOUS

Five months after moving to Brisbane I'm offered work as a flute teacher in Hervey Bay. I pack up my precious belongings, farewell my best friend with more promises of staying in touch, and catch a bus four hours north.

Hervey Bay is hot. Really fucking hot. It's beautiful, sunny, and festooned with the pristine white beaches for which Australia is famous. Elle McPherson and her perfect body debut on our new colour televisions in the Tab Cola commercials. Paul Hogan slips an extra shrimp on the barbie for wannabe tourists. And I'm finally a completely independent adult, legally allowed to drive, vote, and consume alcohol. I launch into my new *career* as a professional flute teacher with much gusto and little clue. I'm just eighteen, and like most newly minted adults, fairly ignorant of my complete and utter ignorance when it comes to the world of being a grown-up.

My flute teaching work has come from a parent keen to get formal tuition for her talented young daughter. She's found another dozen budding young flautists and established a small teaching practice for me. I love it. I don't know a lot but I'm getting started. I've had four years' experience under my father's tutelage, and I've been playing and performing for ten years. I know more than my students and that seems to be enough.

Part of me is shamed by the adage, "*Those who can, do. Those who can't, teach.*" And part of me knows I've found my place in the world.

I'm good at this. I love my students. I take them to the local eisteddfod where they perform quartets from memory, with pretty bows in their hair and polished bows at the end. They win first place. I hire a hall, charge parents $2 entry fee, and put on a concert where every student performs. We all love it. Teaching brings me nothing but satisfaction; there's no performance anxiety or overwhelming doubt at my ability. I'm not consumed with fear about mistakes or judgments. I'm home. I feel like an eighteen-year-old mother to eighteen young people.

Socially, I remain isolated. My circle of students and their families keep me busy, but they're not friends. They're not even peers. I live in a share house with a girl I met briefly, but our lives are busy, and we spend no time together. I know nobody else.

News from home is filled with worry and angst about my sister. She's thirteen years old and no longer attending school, her behaviour erratic. She stares for hours into the night at the television static that appears long after the test screen has ended. It reminds me of the film, *Poltergeist*. "They're he-ere."

The beautiful little girl who faithfully followed her big brother everywhere while quietly sucking her two middle fingers long into her teens, morphs into a screeching banshee. Uncontrollable. Disappearing out the window in the middle of the night. Returned home by the police on more than one occasion. Secretly starting to purge, self-harm, and sleep with an older boyfriend. She declares her career goal to be prostitution in Sydney and runs away from home. She's returned the next day. My mother's enormously distressed, searching for answers and looking for someone to blame. My father valiantly tries all suggestions. He moves out of the family home and into a small flat with Vanessa, enrolling her in the nearby Seventh-Day Adventist school. Nothing changes. They return home after a few months.

Within twelve months, my parents' marriage is falling apart. There's no support for them and they don't know how to support each other. My mother rings me to say life isn't worth living. I don't know how to process this information, but I'm deeply familiar with the desire to not exist. I return for a family therapy session with a Lismore psychiatrist. We sit in a circle and learn about our contributions to Vanessa's unsociable and inexplicable behaviours. Dad isn't strict enough. My mother is too critical. Kristin spends less time with her. And I left home. I don't recall any discussion of Vanessa's contribution to Vanessa's behaviour or useful information for my parents to manage her or support each other.

By 1985, I'm settled in my teaching life but torn between feeling purposeful and purposeless. I love teaching and music and the identity it offers me. Simone the musician. Simone the teacher. But I'm also painfully aware of my social awkwardness, unappealing appearance, inability to make friends, and overwhelming loneliness. I live in paradise, but without friends to enjoy the spectacular Queensland sunrises, I feel bereft.

I'm desperate to be slim and pretty, the ultimate key to success, according to my mother and grandmother. I'm envious of my little sister's effortless beauty and mystified as to why she can't appreciate her natural gifts. My understanding of mental health issues is limited to schizophrenia as demonstrated by Jack Nicholson in *One Flew Over the Cuckoo's Nest*, and dissociative identity disorder from Flora Schreider's *Sybil*. I have no appreciation for the enormous impact depression and anxiety have on our family and have never heard of borderline personality disorder. I come to the erroneous conclusion that Vanessa's a difficult little shit and needs to get her act together. It's a long time before I develop empathy for her, and by then, it's too late. I continue to live with regret at my lack of understanding. Could I have done more?

I confide my fears and feelings to nobody, instead burying my head in fantasy books, numbers, music, and any morsel of food I can afford. I stare at sugary delights with a longing in my soul and pass by the salads with disdain for their commonness. I've learned to shovel food in so quickly, I don't even notice I've eaten it.

I turn nineteen in February 1985. I've been teaching in Hervey Bay for eight months and have maintained my teaching practice but not grown it. Financially, life is a struggle. I have no words or understanding for my intense emotions, continuing to ignore and numb them. My housemate is rarely home but has a large collection of medications she keeps around the house. I have no idea what they are. There's plenty of Panadol, but the rest of the prescription medications are a mystery to me. When she travels away for yet another weekend of festivities, I find every pill in the house and swallow them all. It's a big effort to swallow several hundred pills; there's a lot of water involved and I'm sculling as quickly as my belly will allow. I don't know what I've taken, but I figure quantity over quality should do the job. I want out.

But I'm naive and ignorant and have no idea about medications. I pass out for a day or so and wake up feeling bitter remorse at my inability to do something as simple as kill myself, and panic at how to explain all the missing medications to my housemate. I resolve to say nothing and hope she doesn't notice. An enormous parcel arrives in the post for her, filled with marijuana freshly shipped from Nimbin. She's happy with her delivery and there's never any mention of the missing medications. I move out soon after.

I've never paid much attention to anxiety as a mental health condition or to the panic attacks experienced with out-of-control anxiety. I'm fifty years old before I'm diagnosed with severe generalised anxiety. But I'm nineteen when I have my first panic attack. I don't understand what's happening.

After my failed overdose, I rent a small, comfortable room at Phil's house in Hervey Bay. I adore Phil. She's sixty-five years old, and to my nineteen-year-old self, seems ancient, wise, and comfortable in her own skin. She's the first person to really mother me. My little room has a single wooden bed with a small shelf for books and a reading light in the bedhead. I have a dressing table by my bed and an antique wardrobe to store my clothes. For reasons I no longer recall, I crawl into the dusty wardrobe and sit on the floor trying to stop the flood of tears, slow my breathing, quell the trembling, and get control of myself. I hate crying and emotions. It feels like tangible shame. People don't cry in my family.

I have no idea Phil knows I'm there, but she opens the door and escorts me from the wardrobe, sitting me in a chair with a cup of tea and telling me everything's going to be fine—it's just a bad day. She puts the television on, and we watch *Sale of the Century*. I promptly start answering Tony Barber's questions and watch the divine Delvene Delaney offer gift after gift to each contestant. My heartrate settles and life goes on. We never talk about it again.

The emotional distress of our disintegrating family unit leaves my mother slimming down to a frighteningly small version of herself. We have a very poor relationship, but now that I'm an adult, I want to connect with her in an adult manner. I love musicals, she loves musicals, so we decide to go to Sydney to see the new Andrew Lloyd Webber musical that's just arrived in Australia—*Cats*.

I make the eight-hour trek to Ballina by bus, collect my mother, then we head to Sydney—another excruciating twelve hours along the Pacific Highway, winding through towns coloured with the sights and scents of jacarandas, frangipanis, macadamias, avocados, and the ever-present wattle. Sydney is hot and busy and overrun with people. We spend the night in a hotel and head off to see *Cats*. A Coca Cola can larger than a small car is decorating the front row of the dress circle where we find ourselves seated—the entire theatre transformed into a city alley from a cat's perspective. I've been listening to the music on my record player for months; I know every word by heart. We have a fantastic night together at the theatre before making the twenty-hour trek back to Queensland. I cautiously hope that a new era of mother-daughter bonding is just around the corner.

While living in Hervey Bay, I keep attending flute society events in Brisbane. The head of the Tasmanian Conservatorium of Music chats to me about the possibility of doing a music degree.

"But flute players are a dime a dozen," I say.

"Not good ones," he says. And I'm left wondering if he's paid me a compliment.

THE APOSTLES

How easy it is to love. How hard it is to be loved.

I have beautiful friends. I really do. Amazing, kind, intelligent, supportive, thoughtful, empathetic, giving, honest, creative, awesome people. I don't have a huge circle of friends—nor do I want a lot. Quality over quantity is a philosophy I've matured into.

When I was a wee thing, I only had Friendly. I'm sure this probably bothered me. I don't know; I can't remember. With constant moving from one house to another—new schools all the time—it isn't easy always being the new kid, so I cast a protective shell around myself at a very young age and relied on my invisible friend. But underneath was a fragile little girl who second-guesses everything she sees, hears, says, thinks, and does.

I found amazing friends at university and kept them all these years. They're like sisters, teaching me what my family could not—love, compassion, acceptance, and belonging. Teaching me how to be forgiven for making a mistake and how freeing it is to be honest and vulnerable, even when it scares the crap out of me. I'm here today because of my friends—the old and the new.

I have an unerring need to care for, and protect, anyone who crosses my path, so I'd rather blow a million ridiculous scenarios completely out of proportion in my head than darken a friend's day with my weirdness. I cannot tell an untruth; I won't lie to your face. But I'm an expert at dodging questions, redirecting the conversation, and lying by omission. My ever-patient support crew learn to tease out the facts.

I have undying gratitude to all my friends—near and far—for their faith in me. I hear them cheering from the sidelines, and I may look like my shoulders droop and my gait is slowing, that my resolve waivers, but every cheer lifts my spirit and spurs me a little further along. Lasting change isn't done quickly. It's done by ever so slowly absorbing a new way of being—one painful step at a time.

My crew numbers twelve—like the Apostles who stood by Jesus Christ. My husband, my psychologist, and an eclectic group of ten scattered around the country.

To my circle of beautiful friends and my patient and devoted husband, SHMILY. *See How Much I Love You.*

AND THEN THERE WERE FRIENDS

I enrol into a Bachelor of Music (Performance) at the Tasmanian Conservatorium of Music, apply for a job as a housemistress at a private girl's school in Hobart, and in January 1986, pack up my teaching studio, take the three flights to Tasmania, and start again.

I spend three years at the Tasmanian Conservatorium of Music. I practice regularly, fall in love with ensemble and orchestral playing, and find myself no longer the best player in town. I've been a medium-sized fish in very small ponds for a long time and I'm quickly brought down a peg or two. Near enough is never going to be good enough. Perfection is a must.

In February 1987, I turn twenty-one. It's the year Kylie Minogue bursts into fame with *Locomotion*, Melbourne endures the horror of the Hoddle Street Massacre, and Prime Minister Bob Hawke boldly promises, *no child will live in poverty by 1990*. My birthday is celebrated at Beaujangles restaurant with my mother, her friends visiting from New South Wales and Kerry from my childhood days in Howrah. My fashion sense remains dreadful, not assisted by the puffy sleeves and poofy hair iconic to the '80s, and my inability to see, accept, and work with my body's natural shape and size.

I gain confidence as a flautist but lose confidence as a young woman. I'm a twenty-one-year-old virgin and desperately ashamed of this fact. Invited to a university party hosted by the engineering department, I meet a bearded student who takes the time to talk and flirt with me. The budding engineers have brewed a lethal concoction that tastes like cordial and inebriates like pure ethanol. My natural desire to binge on all things sweet and delicious finds me pretty drunk and tucked up in a single bed with my new bearded friend. I try to hide my complete lack of experience, but he soon figures it out and isn't in the least bit fazed. We liaise a few more times over the next month and I finally feel the shame of being completely undesirable as a woman start to shed a little. It's a few more years before I find a man with whom I'm comfortable to be seen in public, but I indulge in a few more dalliances in the meantime. I still hate everything about my body but discover some men will accept it as is.

In April 1988, the Australian Flute Societies hold their seventh national flute convention in Adelaide. I convince three other flute players at the Conservatorium that they should attend. We bundle into my 1976 bright orange Holden Gemini and drive a gruelling two days from Hobart to Adelaide for the convention. It becomes the first of a great many sojourns we make in my little orange car over the years, as the four of us become the best of friends; I just call them The Girls. We play flute quartets for the sailors on the ferry to Melbourne, meet up with American sailors when a US naval ship comes to town, and eventually drink all the profits from our short-lived catering business.

We still gather together at least once a year for a shopping trip and debrief, and in this era of social media, we chat almost daily. The Girls become not just friends but the sisters I always yearned to have. They share my love of music, along with their own insecurities, fears, hopes, and dreams. They teach me about friendship and forgiveness. Success and failure. And when my life falls apart twenty-five years later, they're a crucial ingredient in the glue that holds me together. I learn a great many things in my three years at the Tasmanian Conservatorium of Music, but the most valuable possession I leave with is true friendship.

As 1988 rolls around, I'm knee-deep in friendships and occasional trysts, while my little sister is sixteen, heavily pregnant and alone. She moves from Ballina to Tasmania to be near me. So does my mother. My parents have separated—unable to reconcile their sorrow and despair with Vanessa's ongoing issues. The baby is due in early April, and I leave Vanessa with strict instructions not to give birth during the four days I'm far away at the flute convention. Her waters break while I'm gone, she goes into labour, and Jamie arrives safe and sound on Friday 01 April. When the phone call comes through that she's had her baby, I think it's an April Fools' Day trick. It's not. I tell dad, and he beams with pride at the news that he's a grandfather.

My mother takes to grandparenthood with unexpected love and gusto. Despite her shame and reservations with the public knowledge of a pregnant teenage daughter, she stands by Vanessa's side throughout the pregnancy and those early newborn days, falling completely in love with Jamie. To her dying day, she yearns to live near her grandchildren, showering them with the love and affection her children so desperately craved.

I leave my job as a housemistress at the boarding school and become a live-in nanny to three rambunctious rapscallions under the age of four. Life gets even busier, but I fall in love with the kids and get on well with their parents. I get to know the family friends as well and feel an even deeper sense of belonging. One morning, I wake to learn the closest friends of my nannying family have lost their only child to SIDS. A healthy eight-month-old baby—dead. Just like my brother.

The grief is palpable; I feel waves of it washing over me, threatening to strip away the carefully constructed façade of strength I've swathed myself in since childhood. I share the news with my mother and receive unexpected sympathy and warmth from her. She knows what it is to lose a child. We attend the funeral together—the first funeral I've ever attended— viewing the tiny white coffin front and centre in the semi-circular church. The emotions are overwhelming, and I have no idea how to deal with them. For the first time in my studies, I ask for an extension on a university essay as I try to process the grief all around me. It's turned down. I stay up all night typing an essay, discovering work to be an effective tool at disguising emotions.

While my fair-skinned, red-headed self is suited to cold climates, my olive-skinned, dark-haired sister is not. Within three months, she can't stand the cold, and jumps on a plane to the Gold Coast with my nephew. My mother soon follows. By the end of the year, both of them are unhealthily slim, and phone calls with each are filled with frustration about the other—my mother constantly worried about Vanessa's erratic behaviour and imperfections, Vanessa irritated by her incessant criticisms that are sometimes valid, sometimes not. Somehow, I'm expected to mediate and reconcile their differences, a role I was cast into as a child and relish as an adult. But in this case, I feel powerless. Phone calls are something to dread, as rarely do they bring anything but bad news and stressful conversations.

My friendship with The Girls grows stronger. I socialise. Party. Have sleepovers. I have what I've always yearned for—a sense of belonging. I don't need my mother or my sister; I relegate them to the back of my mind as a couple of lunatics. But I miss Jamie. I lack understanding or appreciation of mental health issues and the fathomless depths of the parental bond, no matter the flaws of the parent.

By the end of 1988, I have a difficult decision to make. I have an established network of friends, I'm finding teaching and performing work, and I'm well settled in home and university life. But I've lost all respect for the teachers at the Conservatorium and yearn to go elsewhere for my final year. If I'm going to move to another university, it must have the best flute teachers in Australia and I decide on the Canberra School of Music. I mail off a hastily produced audio cassette of my playing, with a scribbled note asking if I have what it takes to get into the school. I'm told I have a good chance, but there's no guarantee until I do a live audition. I withdraw from the Tasmanian Conservatorium, practice for the audition, pack everything I own into the little orange Gemini, and prepare for the two-day drive to the nation's capital, Canberra, taking an almighty leap of faith that I'll get into the prestigious school.

FOOD RULE 08

If I eat today, I can't eat tomorrow.

TRANSITIONS

"**A**re you on a diet?"

Christmas Day 1988. It's hot and summery, cherry trees laden with fruit and bushes overflowing with raspberries, strawberries, and blueberries. The air is deliciously warm with the salty scent of roast meats I have no intention of consuming.

"Umm . . ."

Shit. He can see my fat stomach? Why would he ask that?

Yellow flowers scattered across the brown '70s wallpaper cheerfully mimic five festive faces while my heart pounds a million miles a minute.

"Oh no, dear! His English not so good. He means why you don't eat meat."

My thoughts freeze while my tongue firmly attaches to my gritted teeth. I've never met the Japanese couple before. Like me, they are away from family at a time of year when Australian families traditionally congregate together.

"No!" laughs Kirsten. "She's vegetarian."

We've known each other since we were eleven years old and she's one of The Girls from my Conservatorium friends. But in 1988, my first Christmas away from family, she has no idea I have issues with disordered eating and severe body image problems. Nobody knows—not even me.

We set the table—the familiar act of arranging plates calming my panic while dishes are piled with roast meats and vegetables, salads, sides, and delectable delights. The endless noise in my head rattles on.

What do I eat? They'll notice if I don't eat. Just eat salad? Pile my plate and ignore the diet comment? How fat he must think I am! Japanese people are tiny. I'm the fattest person in the room. I don't want to eat. I want to go to the toilet and hide. I want to go home.

"It was a pig of a thing to wrap."

Kirsten hands me a gift. It's a heavy, irregularly shaped lump of red and white Santas.

"It was such a pig of a thing to wrap."

She's giggling. Everyone's laughing and I'm the butt of some huge joke. Are they making fun of me being a pig? Do they ALL think I'm really fat?

"Go on. Open it!"

I open it with delicate precision, carefully levering sticky tape from jolly little Santas.

"You wouldn't believe what a pig of a thing it was to wrap."

I unwrap a sleeping concrete pig—his little piggy tail tucked under a chubby little bottom. The perfect garden ornament. The room fills with fits of laughter. It's gorgeous. I love it and finally get the pig-of-a-thing-to-wrap joke. Now I'm with the in-crowd. Pig survives twenty years until too many chips from my careless kids mean I finally say goodbye to another piece of my youth.

I go home from my first Christmas at a friend's house feeling simultaneously loved and cared for and hideously upset with my food consumption and weight. *Are you on a diet?* echoing through my head well into the New Year. I'm always on a diet, trying to change my weight.

My *weight*.

Age twenty-two, my weight is now the healthiest it's ever been. I'm not yet—and have never been—an overweight adult. Within twelve months, I'm bulimic.

As I leave my little share house in Sandy Bay a few weeks after Christmas, The Girls come over to say farewell. We all hug goodbye, promise to stay in touch, and as I drive off, I see them in my rear vision mirror waving goodbye. They are true to their word. I still have more than twenty-five handwritten letters detailing the ebbs and flows, triumphs and tragedies of post-university life as we gradually disperse around the country in search of careers, partners, and purpose. Our bonds of friendship grow stronger despite time and distance.

The eight years I spend in Canberra, freezing my butt off in winter and oozing sweat through summer, mark my transition from student to professional. Single and carefree, to married and earth mother. Slender to fat. Problematic eating to bulimic. Eight transitional years filled with performance on stage and radio, in theatres and gardens, solos, chamber music, and orchestras. Romance, friendship, mentors, and mentees. Success, failure, confidence, anxiety, grief, elation. Weddings, funerals, miscarriage, orgasms. These years are busy and full, and there's no time to sit around contemplating my feelings or wondering why I am as I am.

It's mid-summer when I arrive, my little orange car surviving the exhausting two-day drive, packed to the brim with precious belongings. I answer the first ad I see for a boarder, studiously practice until my allotted audition time, and try to get a feel for living in the nation's capital—the first place I've ever lived not by the ocean. The trees grow in straight lines. I don't like it.

My audition is successful. Far from perfect, as my grandmother would say, but adequate enough to be admitted into the Canberra School of Music. Given my backup plan doesn't exist, this is fortunate. Changing from one tertiary institution to another means the curriculum is different and standards vary, so my final year takes two years as I have to catch up with some theoretical subjects.

Finally, I've arrived at the big pond. I've played the flute for fifteen years and have always been one of the better players around, but until now, I've lived in pretty small ponds. I'm in with the big fry and my true ability, tenacity, and work ethic are about to be tested. I have the teachers of my dreams—mentors I look up to. Flautists I want to equal. Teachers who inspire with words and actions. Students who inspire with talent and commitment.

The move to the Canberra School of Music turns out to be a very good move indeed. My practice time doubles, and ensemble opportunities triple. I find ample private teaching and soon find myself ensconced in the local musical community, mentoring at the Canberra Youth Orchestra, volunteering with the Canberra Flute Society, and performing at weddings, funerals, Parliament House, embassies, galas, conventions, and festivals. I feel a deep sense of belonging in the musical community.

Once again, my public life is in deep contrast to my private life. When I'm with other people, I pull on my big girl panties and play the role of confident, competent, personable, reliable, and responsible Simone. When I close my door and I'm alone, the overwhelming dread at my inadequacy and the fear that nothing I do will ever be good enough consumes me. I try not to think. I try not to eat. The more I think about not thinking and eating, the more I think and eat. My secret world of hidden eating shames me, but after twenty years, it's safe and familiar.

I move into a large group home and develop a strong and lasting friendship with Emma—my fellow redhead. One of our flatmates names us the Two Botticellis—pale skin and heads crowned with thick golden locks. My fellow Botticelli is tiny; I feel monstrous by comparison. When our unruly large group house becomes too much, Emma, her partner, and I move into a much smaller group home where I make more close friends. I feel part of a family—a connection to peers who are warm and demonstrative, creative and artistic. I love our house full of happy, creative, university students. I learn to accept and receive hugs—something completely foreign to me. I learn to feel accepted and wanted—something I've yearned for. I learn to stick my fingers down my throat and purge.

I practice and rehearse at least six hours a day, take long brisk walks to burn calories, and visit the gym where I swim for an hour, then wander around equipment, feeling overwhelmed, stupid, and enormous. I do aerobic classes and hate my F cup breasts and their refusal to be contained in the beige monstrosities that are the only options available in the larger section of the lingerie department.

I'm living a juxtaposition of the happiest years of my life while sinking ever deeper into a pit of self-hatred. The puppy fat grandma talked of all those years ago is a shadow I can't shake. No matter the number on the scales or the dress tag, all I see is plump. Big boobs. Big hips. Big girl. And big is bad. I've become terrified of men and had no intimate connections since a shameful one-night stand with a married sailor on the ferry from Hobart to Melbourne enroute to Canberra. My mother decides I must be a lesbian, because I've never had a boyfriend and never shared news of my dalliances with her.

BULIMIA

Salty tears stream down my face, landing on the corners of my lips before dripping off my chin. The deep magenta flush glowing on my cheeks a stark contrast to the enormous grey circles appearing beneath my reddened eyes.

My housemates sit around the dining table laughing with our dinner guests. The remains of our meal spread across the table, our scattered empty wine bottles witnessing the ever-increasing volume as tales of wit, wisdom, and woe from the day are shared with great gusto and exaggeration.

Emma and I spent the afternoon preparing heaped platters of spaghetti and a Greek salad with enormous chunks of salty feta and generous portions of olives, which I carefully extract and set to the side of my plate. Fresh loaves of bread from the local bakery complete the meal spread across the old pine desk with its three small drawers that serves as our dining table.

The room is awash with friendship and a sense of sharing that goes far beyond the helpings of spaghetti. We're an eclectic group of university students—musician, sculptor, writer, and fashion designer—brought together by an economic need to share living costs, but staying together because we fell in love with each other's company.

Two glasses of wine go straight to my head before moving south to my bladder, with its irrepressible need to evacuate contents constantly and urgently. Topics of conversation from that evening have long since passed from easy recall, but gut-piercing laughter and a sense of oneness with humanity are etched deep into my heart.

"You look like an Afghan dog!" someone guffaws, as my uncontrollable laughter at an unexpected moment leaves me dribbling wine down my chin, my waist-length, strawberry blonde hair, wild and loose, hiding my face. The merriment continues from everyone as a little knot of despair starts knocking on the pit of shame nestled in my belly.

I make my way to the toilet and think, *this is it*. I've thought about it a lot but never before tried it. This time it's different.

I lift the toilet seat, freshly cleaned that day for our dinner party, and stare at the shiny white porcelain. I tuck my hair into the back of my shirt, bend over, and push my fingers to the back of my throat in search of the automatic gag reflex, regretting the long fingernails I've valiantly tried to grow. My stomach heaves, but nothing happens. I remove my fingers and take a deep breath, feeling the warm air fill my belly. I bend over and try again. It takes several attempts, but finally long strands of barely chewed and undigested spaghetti start to come up. I've crossed a line and there's no turning back. This is who I am now.

Time slows and stops. My thick frizzy hair struggles to be contained, but my hand becomes an expert at forcing the recently devoured meal back, spaghetti stretching the length of my oesophagus as I pull individual strands all the way out. Soon the porcelain bowl is filled with the meal lovingly prepared only a few hours previously. The two fingers that laboured to retrieve the contents now indented with teeth marks. I stand. Stretch. Hold my shoulders back. Soggy toilet paper sticks to my fingers in little clumps like the patches on Australian television personality Norman Gunston's shaving nicks, as I endeavour to wipe the digestive slime away. I have no thought or care for the physical consequences; I've never had any respect for my unlovable body, and this feels no different. If it leads me to a happy weight, to hell with the consequences.

I straighten my skirt, rub my eyes, clean my hand again, then flush the toilet—ensuring no evidence remains once the water has settled. The old 1960s bathroom is adjacent to the toilet with its ancient porcelain sink and lemon-yellow bath. I close the door, wash my hands thoroughly, rinse my mouth, and inspect my face in the mirror.

I look into my watery eyes to see if anything's changed. I look just the same but everything's different now. The exhaustion of vomiting is spreading through my body while the exhilaration of an empty stomach is giving me a rush of endorphins. Finally, I've found a way to have my cake and eat it too. Finally, I know how to control my weight.

The table of congeniality barely notices as I slip back into my pine dining chair. I pick up my glass, swirl the smooth red wine around in my mouth, and wash away the last remnants of the purged meal. Everything is the same as before. But everything has changed.

The last months of 1990 roll into a blur and purging becomes a normal part of my daily routine, every compliment about my disappearing waistline another confirmation that I'm doing the right thing. My university days are coming to a heady end.

My Bachelor of Music in Performance culminates with a graduation recital in Llewellyn Hall at the Canberra School of Music. It's a big deal, and for a big deal, I need a great frock. I go clothes shopping with Emma and our fashion designer housemate, and after much angst, purchase a strapless black velvet Laura Ashley ball gown. It's gorgeous. I feel like a princess, and with my escalation of purging, starving, and exercising, find the size ten dress needs last-minute alterations to keep it perched above the nipple line.

The hall seats 1,300; there's no way I'll fill it, nor would I expect to. I advertise and invite friends, family, teachers, students, and my fellow flautists. My parents make the 1,000-kilometre trek down by bus from Ballina. Several hundred people come to see me play and I put on the performance I've worked so hard to achieve, performing the music I love—Bach, Feld, Crumb, Briccialdi, Debussy. At the end of the recital, my father comes to the stage and presents me with an enormous bunch of pink and white lilies. I still have a precious, faded photo—my father looking up at me with a look of tremendous pride on his face. I'm overwhelmed with gratitude and love and the exhilaration of performance, mixed with the all too familiar, *Thank Christ that's over!*

Part of me is glad my parents separated; I naturally want both of them to be happy, and if that happiness is best found when apart, well so be it. But part of me still yearns for the illusion of happily-ever-afters in our broken family unit. Having both my parents visiting for my recital is a little bubble of pretend, but when my mother tells Emma what a clever girl she is for someone so short, the little bubble bursts, and I remember our family is bat-shit crazy and we're all happiest in our own little spaces. I'm glad my parents have their own safe spaces.

Life as a student comes to an end. As does our group house. Emma and her partner want to move out on their own. I make plans to travel to South America post-university, carefully saving all my teaching money and purchasing a one-way ticket to Guatemala.

I move into a giant, subsidised, twelve-bedroom group house until it's time to fly away. I've finished studying, but I'm fully immersed in the Canberra musical world—teaching ninety students during the week, performing in chamber music groups weekends and evenings, and invited to big orchestral spectaculars in different parts of New South Wales from time to time. I start doing professional auditions and wonder if perhaps I'll realise my childhood dream and make it as an orchestral flute player. I don't realise it at the time, but these are the glory days of my musical career.

FOOD RULE 13

Only consume liquids.

BONES

I move into the new group house in February 1991 and meet Michael who kindly helps me up the stairwell with the furniture. He's skinny and bald and I barely notice him, but I'm grateful when he offers to put my double bed together. He tells one of the housemates he wants to be sure it's put together properly; he has a thing for redheads and likes the way I look.

This group house is very different from my previous experiences; everyone does their own thing and has an individual cupboard and spot in the kitchen. The bathrooms are like public toilet facilities. With so many people in the house, personnel changes all the time—but Michael is a constant.

Not long after I move in, he ends the relationship with his girlfriend. We start chatting in the evenings and I learn he's recovering from alcohol and drug addiction. He prefers to be called Mick—most of his friends call him Bones—and he loves old Holden cars.

His world is a million miles away from mine. He's ex-military and working as a mechanic. He's intelligent, honest, and loyal. He's opinionated, brash, and unapologetic. The most he knows about music is how to fix the stereo and all the words to Pink Floyd's *Another Brick in the Wall*. But as the months go by, I find myself looking out for his old pink and cream HR ute—aptly named The Pig—when I come home each day. I stay up late to watch television, just because he's there. We hang with other housemates and go to the movies as a group. Then just on our own. There's a deepening connection between us, yet he says and does nothing, so I wonder if I'm misreading things. I'm desperately inexperienced in the world of dating and I don't know what to do.

The Girls and I stay in contact and catch up whenever we can. Tuesday, 02 July 1991, Kirsten and I plan a trip to Melbourne in my faithful old Gemini to meet the others for a week filled with too much gin, cake ogling, and a trip to the ballet. The night before driving from Canberra to Melbourne I head to bed late, then change my mind. It's been four months; I'm sick of waiting.

I gather my pitiful courage, knock on Mick's door, and say, "I don't want to sleep alone tonight."

He takes my hand, and we head back to my bedroom with the sturdy double bed and a box of condoms. It's a night like no other. This time, I'm with a guy I care about. This time, we know each other before having sex. This time, I'm with someone that cares about me.

It's a long night with little sleep before waking early for the seven-hour drive to Melbourne. I soon tell Kirsten about my night with Mick. We chat about men, relationships, and sex right up until my car blows a tyre—another first. One minute, we're driving down the freeway at 100 kilometres per hour, chatting about boys, and the next, there's a huge bang and the car veers off the road. It's fortunate we didn't hit anything or lose control. A kindly stranger pulls over and helps us change the destroyed tyre for the spare, then we continue, driving a lot more cautiously.

Usually trips away with The Girls are joyous times where I feel a deep connection, soaking up every moment and not wanting it to end. This time, I can't wait to go home. A little piece of my heart has been made vulnerable and it's waiting back in Canberra. There are no mobile phones or internet, so Mick and I don't communicate until I return home a week later. We pick up right where we left off.

I'm twenty-five, and I finally have a boyfriend. A real one. A man I walk around in public with, hand-in-hand. We're young and full of vim and libido. I feel a sense of normality; I'm a normal girl, with a normal boy, and now society can accept me. Now a *man* accepts me. Just as I am. This was the dream from ten years ago and I'd almost given up hope. Yet here he was—my knight in oil-stained armour.

I don't know how to feel about my adult body. Nobody has ever seen it naked before, earlier dalliances half-dressed or covered in bedding. But Mick revels in my curves, and I allow him to see me—still uncomfortable in my own skin but appreciative that someone can find me attractive. I finally experience an orgasm with a man and realise what all the fuss is about. I'm blissfully content. We seem an odd couple, with my background in classical music, tertiary education, vegetarianism, and being a good girl, and his, in stark contrast to mine, a background in helicopters, motorcycles, addiction, and being a bad boy. But I'm attracted to his obvious intelligence, honesty, loyalty, resilience, strength, and brash confidence. He's put a little crack in the armour I've plastered around my vulnerable essence, and I feel an unfamiliar deep sense of trust in another human being. We share similar world views with a passion to care for those who can't care for themselves and to look after the environment.

I agree to start eating chicken; he agrees to start eating vegetables. I still throw up all my food, and nobody has any idea; I certainly have no intention of sharing this secret with the one man that has finally accepted me. I'm well known for my overactive bladder, so extra trips to the bathroom aren't noticed by anybody. I always double check the toilet to ensure everything is properly flushed. I've never had such clean toilets. It's my secret shame, and I'm convinced I can never control my weight in any other manner. When I'm around others, I'll eat food, but when I'm on my own, I only have soups and smoothies. I read it in a book somewhere—the liquid diet. It's going to solve all my problems. It doesn't.

I ask Mick if he'll come to Guatemala, but he can't; he's just started a new job. We decide we'll go together later, so I sell my ticket. I've still never been to South America. In December, we move into our first house together—a gorgeous little weatherboard cottage on the slopes of Mount Ainslie with a wild overgrown garden and ancient blood red roses with a sweet, heady scent. The house rarely catches a glimpse of sunshine, but the beauty of the wild garden and the proximity to Mount Ainslie and its wealth of kangaroos and kookaburras makes it a perfect haven. We travel to northern New South Wales to meet my parents, both of whom are happy in their new relationships. Dad and Mick chat about motorcycles and politics and enjoy each other's company. My mother says, "I thought you'd find someone more artistic."

By February 1992, my sister is out-of-control, in and out of psychiatric hospitals against her will, diagnosed with borderline personality disorder, on psychiatric medications that don't work, and attempting suicide on a regular basis—cutting, overdosing, setting her house on fire. After the fourth attempt, she ends up in a coma for a few days, so dad asks if my four-year-old nephew can come and live with me until Vanessa is more stable. Of course, I say yes. Mick and I have lived together for three months, and now we're raising a young child. We're a family.

I become Jamie's legal guardian and enrol him into kindergarten. He isn't my biological child, but I take to motherhood like a duck to water. I don't know what I'm doing when thrust into parenthood with a child needing the extra care and attention any child would when abandoned by both parents. But his nature is laid back and friendly. We muddle through the muddy waters and love him to bits. I still dread the telephone, wondering if the next call will be the one to say Vanessa is dead. The call doesn't come.

WILL YOU MARRY ME?

On 01 July 1992, I'm watching television in the evening, the blazing open fire keeping us snug and warm from the freezing Canberra nights. I'm in an old pair of over-sized pyjamas and look like a train wreck at the end of the day.

Mick comes in wearing boxer shorts, kneels down, takes my hand, and looks up with his keenly intelligent blue eyes. "Will you marry me?"

I start laughing, thinking it's a joke. We've had many discussions about marriage, and he's always disparaged the idea as an unnecessary societal construct leftover from a patriarchal society.

"Will you marry me?"

He's serious. *Oh my God! Of course, yes!* There's no ring or romantic gestures; we struggle financially, and Mick is far more practical than he will ever be romantic. It's non-traditional, but it doesn't matter. This is definitely the man I want to be with; I feel a deep knowing of certainty in the depths of my belly. It's not just the lustful love of youth; we have a strong intellectual connection, a powerful friendship, and an innate sense of trust in each other. I can barely contain myself and want to tell all my friends, but it's late, so I have to wait. I'm the last of my friends to find a partner and the first to be betrothed. We set a date—Sunday, 13 December 1992.

The next six months pass in a flurry of activity. We both work full-time at odd hours, and we're raising my sister's four-year-old child, living the mundane realities of running a home and have a wedding to plan. There's just one thing I need to get off my chest before the big day. I want our marriage to begin with complete openness, so I arrange a babysitter for Jamie and we go to dinner at our favourite Turkish restaurant, replete with giant floor cushions and a red-headed belly dancer.

"There's something I want to tell you," I say, once the dips and breads are brought to the table. "This is really hard for me to say but with your history of twelve-step recovery, I'm hoping you understand."

We sit in silence as he waits for me to continue, but I don't know where to start. Patience and long pauses are something he's good at, so he just waits for me to gather my thoughts and courage.

"I'm bulimic."

Twenty-eight years later, I have vivid recall of the restaurant: the leather motorcycle jacket Mick was wearing, the blue tablecloth, along with the pounding of my heart and the grip of anxiety at the back of my throat. But I have no recollection of the rest of the conversation. Sharing the shame with someone I trusted implicitly was enough to settle my nerves, let go of the fear, and brave the next conversation.

"Also, while I'm sharing all the skeletons in my closet, I took an overdose when I was nineteen."

The rest of the evening disappears into the cavernous recesses of lost memories, for both of us. Mick had no idea what bulimia was, I offered no more information, and he didn't ask—a pattern of communication that continued for many years to come. My purging went unnoticed a couple more years before I decided enough was enough. Mick—never renowned for his Sherlock Holmes level of observation—first learned of my purging when I was admitted to a psychiatric hospital twenty-four years later.

Sharing two of the most shameful secrets of my life doesn't have a lasting impact on him. Nor does it impact our decision to marry. At 10 a.m. on Sunday, 13 December 1992, I send Mick's younger brother out to redirect any wedding guests we've been unable to contact regarding the eleventh-hour change of venue. The heavens have unexpectedly opened, and flood rain is cascading down at our outdoor bush wedding. We move to plan B—the community centre at Corroboree Park in Ainslie.

Mick spends the morning pretending nothing unusual is happening and proceeds to trim branches off wattle trees with a chainsaw. I spend the morning in a panic of obsessive organisation. By the time we get to Corroboree Park, I've arranged all the flowers, food, and drink in the little hall for the reception, gone over the last-minute plans with our celebrant, and ensured Jamie looks adorable in his bow tie as our ring bearer. Mick's finally forced to acknowledge the emotional component of the day, and promptly falls apart, sobbing on friends' shoulders, and leaving me completely alarmed. I count threes in my head.

It's the most simple and economical of weddings. I wear a green skirt and top made by a close friend. The fruitcakes are made by my mother-in-law and decorated by Emma and her partner, awash with fresh rose petals surreptitiously snipped from neighbouring houses in the middle of the night. The wedding flowers are sourced from a wholesaler and arranged beautifully by my mother, and the light afternoon tea is prepared by friends. My flower girls are a student and her sisters, and we all hold bunches of white lilies, the food tables in the hall adorned with white tablecloths and blue cornflowers.

As the ceremony is about to start, clouds clear; the hot summer sun shines on wet glistening leaves and we say our vows under the gum trees, surrounded by a small circle of family and friends. There's nothing elaborate or fancy, but every word is heartfelt and genuine. Public declarations of love and commitment don't come naturally to either of us, but the significance of the moment isn't lost on us. Everything about it feels right.

The day goes off without a hitch. We bundle into my aging Gemini, freshly sprayed with shaving cream and decorated with streamers, and head off on our honeymoon—driving seven hours to Melbourne to catch the ferry to Tasmania for a two-week holiday while dad and his new wife look after Jamie at home. We're ready to begin a whole new chapter of our lives, together.

AN OLD SOUL

The next four years race by in a flurry of teaching, performing, unemployment, reemployment, pregnancy, miscarriage, pregnancy, babies, and sex. Libidos living out their last days with gusto and glee. Dalliances in the forest, by a stream, in the back of a ute by the light of a full moon. Floors, beds, baths, sofas, and kitchen tables. We try a little of everything and let passion devour one another each and every day.

In January 1994, Jamie returns to his mother. He's almost six years old and lived with us for nearly two years. Our quirky little instant family thrust together under strange and difficult circumstances, coming to an end just before Mick and I enter into parenthood the traditional way, with the birth of our first child. Sending Jamie back is heartbreaking. Is it the right thing to do? Should we have sent him back? I don't know. I'll never know if it was the right decision for him, given all that transpires over the next two decades. We have a little six-year-old boy who loves us dearly but desperately wants to return to his mother—to care for her as he's always done. So, dad and his wife make the long train trip from Ballina to Canberra, collect Jamie, and return him to Vanessa. I'm six months pregnant. I cry for two months.

My weight slowly creeps up as Mick and I settle into marriage and instant parenthood. No longer am I slim and fit—a joy I experienced just fleetingly in the last years of university. Now I'm a slightly plump woman carrying that puppy fat grandma always talked about. By the twelve-week mark of my first pregnancy, I've gained fifteen kilos. Without a pre-pregnancy weigh-in, it's a statistic I can't prove at my first obstetrics appointment. By the end of the pregnancy, I'll gain thirty-eight kilos.

Sure, I'm eating for two, but it's pretty clear that most of the weight isn't from my baby or placenta, or even flab. I have pre-eclampsia—escalating high blood pressure, protein in my urine, and fluid retention. The puffiness in my legs, hands, and face is a horror to behold. My mother's husband says I look like TVs Auntie Jack. I throw that maternity dress away. The doctor declares me unwell and sends me to the hospital when I'm thirty-five weeks pregnant. I spend two weeks flat on my back with nurses endlessly repeating, *Relax and take it easy*, every time my blood pressure jumps another number. Despite the fact that relaxation doesn't come naturally, I think I'm doing a jolly good job just lying there doing nothing; I'm confused about how to relax more. When my blood pressure tops the 200 mark three weeks before my due date, the doctor says in no uncertain terms, "We've got to get this baby out." And they do.

At 8 a.m. on Sunday, 17 March 1994, I deliver a beautiful, healthy baby boy by caesarean section. He's the first Saint Patrick's Day boy, so all the nurses are pushing us to name him Patrick, but long before we'd conceived, the decision to name our first son had been made. Conor. From the movie *Highlander* where Connor McCloud of Clan McCloud turns out to be quite the immortal hero. Our concession to Saint Patrick's Day is the Irish spelling of Conor—just one N.

My dreams of a natural birth through the birthing centre all evaporate the moment medical problems arise. I've failed my baby and femininity by not delivering naturally—something women never fail to remind me in decades to come. I'm determined to breastfeed. My breasts swell from their pregnancy F cup to an unidentifiable engorged horror I can't bear to look at. But my baby doesn't care. He latches on and suckles with ease. Finally, my body behaves in a way it's designed to do.

It's more than a year since I last purged, and while the thought crosses my mind as my overweight, puffed up body and its gargantuan breasts seem to be on display every time my child is hungry, I decide being fat is better than depleting my body of the nourishment my baby needs. I instinctively protect my children in a way I have never protected my body.

At the moment of delivery, my sky-high blood pressure plummets to normal, but as normal is something my body forgot over the past three months, I'm suffering the physical effects of low blood pressure—constant lightheadedness and feeling that I'm going to pass out. Conor and I stay in hospital another ten days, and then finally, our new family unit goes home.

For the first—and only—time in our marriage, Mick drives sedately. He's as deeply in love with our new son as I am and instinctively protective of us both. We drive at or below the speed limit, no hard braking and acceleration, and no rage at the apparent idiocy of every other motorist on the road. I dream it's the beginning of a new motoring era in our lives. It turns out to be a one-day anomaly.

We arrive home and take a million photos of our precious baby—and a video or two. On one video, I proudly declare I've lost twenty kilos in ten days. It's the second-best thing that's happened in ten days. The other eighteen kilos stubbornly cling to every inch of my body and refuse to depart. I refuse to acknowledge my increasingly sedentary lifestyle— mimicking my husband's natural inclination to sit down a lot—and secret eating that I barely remember and cannot comprehend. It's almost dissociative and as much a secret to me as anyone else. I stop purging soon after we marry, but binging remains a lifelong issue.

My mother and her new husband arrive shortly before Conor's born. She's desperate to spend as much time with her new grandson as possible. They rent a house in the neighbouring suburb and spend quality time getting to know my beautiful baby boy with his old soul and flawless skin.

FOOD RULE 21

Only eat vegetables.

EARTH MOTHER

L ife's good. I've been mothering flute students for a decade, but now I have a real baby to call my own.

"You grow beautiful tomatoes, Mick, but look what I can grow!"

I have almost 100 flute students. I'm highly active in the Canberra Flute Society and Director of the 9th Australian Flute Convention. I'm a tutor for the Youth Orchestra and perform chamber music several nights a week and most weekends. Music makes me whole.

Motherhood brings me home.

I'm called earth mother by the girls in my mother's group. But I confess, it's easy to be earth mother to an easy baby. Conor sleeps midnight to 5 a.m. the day he's born and never looks back. He suckles eagerly, sleeps enthusiastically, and smiles effortlessly. He is, to all intents and purpose, a very easy baby. He's so laid back, I have to wake him up to feed. He's a stark contrast to his brother.

In August 1996, I'm a week overdue when I go into labour. I'm excited because this time I'm determined to deliver naturally. I don't have pre-eclampsia, but I do have the internet, and I've found every article and infographic available on Yahoo Search. Vaginal birth after caesarean is my most popular search term.

My baby doesn't agree. I spend twenty-four hours in the very early stages of labour. Doctors send me off for an x-ray which shows my baby is over 5kg and a face presentation. I'm perfectly safe to keep labouring along, but zero centimetres dilated. "This baby isn't coming out the natural way," they declare. I accept the inevitable, give up on labouring, and have a second caesarean.

Liam is the fattest baby I've ever seen. He has a head of snow-white curls, big pudgy rolls of puppy fat from head to toe, and blue eyes betraying an astonishing intelligence. He hasn't read the book on how to be a good baby.

The nurses keep poking him with needles to test for diabetes. He doesn't have diabetes—he's just fat. He looks abundantly healthy, but my instincts are screaming—he's delicate and fragile. His porcelain white skin burns in the shade on scorching Canberra summer days. Liam's rolls of fat bother my mother enormously—*Stop feeding him so often!*—but I've read again and again that you can't overfeed a breastfed baby, so I let my hungry little boy feed as he much as he needs. His beautiful soft curls nestle into my arm as his little hands reach across my body, touching with unconditional love, oblivious to my size.

Much to my doctor's distress, I refuse to vaccinate him on schedule. We're three months late when we start—no triple antigens, just protection from one disease at a time. He reacts to every single vaccine, and I feel justified in the delay. I'll vaccinate my child—I understand the necessity for herd immunity—but on my schedule, because I won't sacrifice him for the herd. By the time Liam starts school, he's fully vaccinated. My little boy with the head full of golden curls is fiercely independent, highly intelligent, utterly fearless, and highly curious. I see myself reflected in his chubby white cheeks.

I've added another 10kg to the 15kg I retained after Conor's birth. I'm disgusted by my fat and simultaneously content. Music and motherhood work for me, and I work for them. I'm impervious to the incongruous juxtaposition of loving my husband and children unconditionally, with no care in the world for their size, weight, or appearance, while simultaneously feeling disgust at my own body. I want my boys to be happy and healthy in themselves, so I never comment on appearance—theirs or mine—in earshot. In fact, I rarely comment on my appearance to anyone. My self-loathing is a secret. It's my shame to keep.

We're pretty much penniless and live in government-supported housing. We have three bedrooms too small to swing a non-existent cat, on a block big enough to house a herd of hippos. Our dusty backyard is filled with prickly bindiis, rusty old Holden cars, and fat, juicy oxheart tomatoes.

Mick has a passion and talent for tinkering in his sheds and growing edible delicacies. Our yard has garden beds overflowing with a prolific array of tomatoes, zucchinis, onions, garlic, parsley, artichokes, apples, and enough basil to start a basil shop. I decide vegetables are healthy and try to leave all other food groups out of my diet. My new food rule goes the way of all the others. Our lack of financial security rarely bothers me. Money isn't a motivator, and I have things money could never buy—things I'd barely dared to dream would come true. I have my very own little family.

It's 1997, and Mick's out of work again. His military training was excellent for the military but is not useful for procuring permanent work in the civilian world. He decides to study a Diploma in Communications Engineering, and I decide it won't be in Canberra. We pack all our belongings and two little babies into two old cars and a trailer with a hastily constructed and highly irregular wall and roof, then traipse 1,400 exhausting kilometres, across the Bass Strait to Hobart. No money, no jobs, and no prospects, but wads of faith, hope, and love.

Canberra was only ever intended as a stepping-stone in my musical career, but I've stayed seven years. I find a deep sense of purpose and satisfaction in my musical performance and teaching career. Learn how to love and be loved. Gain a husband and two little boys. And hone my eating disorder skills—deep-rooted depression and anxiety simmering away since childhood now buried so far down it's like they don't exist. I have no idea they're there. Canberra is good to me but it's a long way from the ocean, trees are unnaturally neat and tidy, the magpies swoop and attack, and it's really fucking hot. I yearn for the one city that always feels like home—Hobart. It's the fourth time I move here.

Hobart is delightfully cool on the shores of the Derwent River, abounds in natural beauty at the base of Mount Wellington, and in the late '90s is still a very affordable Australian city. Mick enrols with TAFE, and we hope for the best. Hobart isn't kind to my musical career. I'm immersed in the day-to-day energies of raising toddlers on our non-existent income and naively assume my experience as a flautist and teacher in Canberra will be welcomed in Hobart. I've never applied for jobs before, and I suck at it. Simmering anxiety may sit unnoticed in my belly but rears its ugly head at the most inconvenient moments. I find my weight escalating at an alarming rate—in no small part due to the fact that I eat too much and never exercise.

Conor is a breeze. He's labelled intelligent, empathetic, easygoing, and laid back. So laid back, we nickname him Dory when *Finding Nemo* bursts into motion picture fame. So easygoing, we have to teach him to look us in the eye and repeat instructions to ensure he remembers anything at all.

Liam is the personification of independence; I blame Mick, but really, he gets it from me. A mirrored reflection of Conor, Liam walks early and talks late. Early in his talking career, he sits upon my great aunt's knee and declares, *I's the boss.* He hasn't cracked two years of age yet, but it's a prophetic statement; nobody tells Liam what to do. My boys play together beautifully. When Liam's speech is difficult to understand, Conor interprets; he always understands him. I've heard of sibling rivalry, but haven't witnessed it. Yet.

Mick obtains his diploma, and just as our third baby is about to arrive, he's offered work by a friend's husband—a very Tasmanian way to find employment. Having survived two years on AUSTUDY, even a weekly salary below minimum wage is a veritable fortune. A new era dawns.

My childbearing days end when a tubal ligation is performed simultaneously to my third caesarean. After seventy-two hours of full labour pains, the emergency surgery becomes a memorable affair, with the assistant surgeon being scraped off the floor by a nurse after he passes out and the phone ringing in the theatre several times asking the obstetrician to attend a patient in the emergency department. I'm grateful he hangs around to finish my surgery first. Hamish squeezes in at just under ten pounds—my smallest baby. As I'm wheeled away from theatre, he's secure in my arms and latched onto my breast. He's healthy and I'm happy.

ONENESS WITH THE WORLD

L ife's rosy. Sure, money's a struggle, Mick's insistence on overtaking every car on the road is a regular source of friction, and having three kids is naturally exhausting. But I feel life's blessings raining upon me.

I started teaching flute students in 1981. By 1999, I'm pretty good at it and raising kids is just another type of teaching. I look for their individuality and work with it. Liam tries to become a problem solver at an early age. I lie six-week-old Hamish down on a sheepskin, naked in a patch of sunlight for a few minutes—soaking up Tasmania's precious vitamin D as days get shorter and nights get longer. When he starts to cry and disturbs the boys' television viewing of *The Wiggles* and their hot potatoes, Liam stomps on Hamish's belly to try and stop the noise. The noise escalates. I feel a rare moment of pure anger as fear for my newborn surges through me. I grab Liam and smack his little butt—an action in total contradiction to everything I believe in. Now I have fear and guilt. And two screaming babies.

Mick's working life has always meant early mornings and early homecomings which gifts us the opportunity for him to be a hands-on dad. We're in conflict, however, over discipline. My pacifist upbringing and highly sensitive nature yearn for compassion, not violence. Mick's strict Catholic upbringing demands obedience and respect from people I consider too little to understand. But when my way doesn't work, Mick always steps in. Liam prefers to set his own bedtime, and every evening, he toddles out from the wallpapered room with the blue skies and white clouds, only to be promptly returned by his father. I curl up on the couch reading with Conor and nursing Hamish, while Mick takes to lying in bed with our screaming toddler, holding him firm with one arm until eventually exhausted, Liam falls asleep. It takes just a week before, finally, after another night's screaming, he lifts his golden curls up from the pillow and stares at Mick with tear-stained blue eyes saying, *you go now*. He never screams himself to sleep again.

A precious photo now sits in my lounge room. The old marble steps ascend—piled with dirt, autumn leaves, and gravel, tufts of grass erupting along the sides. The woman sits on the edge of the step, dark sunglasses covering her face and a cascade of thick frizzy hair wrapped around her like a cloak. She gazes at the young baby snug at her breast, his hand resting gently on her chest as the nourishing warmth of the milk replenishes his belly.

Wrapped in a cream woollen jacket and fleecy navy pants, his pale bare head the only flesh exposed to the elements. His older brother with the golden curls and rosy red lips leans into her shoulder as he looks out upon the vista, the thoughts in his head a mystery as he clasps chubby toddler hands together around his fleecy yellow tracksuit.

The steps are set in the Hobart Botanical Gardens, with its hilly greenery, giant flower clock, and miniature Japanese gardens. It's 1999 and the world is awash with the fear of an apocalyptic Y2K ending when midnight strikes on December 2000. Will the computers of the world cope with the turn of a new century? My family is complete. Three cherished babies of my own—fat and snuggly and healthy.

Mick and five-year-old Conor stand behind the camera, watching the break in our tour of the gardens. My mother has just flown home after visiting for Hamish's birth. Her words, "All my children have been a tremendous disappointment to me," still ringing in my ears. I can't make sense of her need to say it when I arrive home from the hospital, my precious newborn in my arms. I don't miss her when she leaves.

My sense of oneness in the world is complete. I'm a mother. I'm at peace with the role and can't smother my babies with enough cuddles and kisses—giving them everything I'd yearned for as a child. We're poor, but that's okay. Mick finally has a permanent job and financial security looks to be just a stepping-stone away. But we're filled with the wealth of love and family and the business of raising three boisterous little men.

My body image is in stark contrast to my peaceful soul. I hate it. I'm fat. There's no other word for it. Fat. The ginormous breasts my mother suggested I have reduced seventeen years prior, engorged with the life-giving milk nourishing my baby. I'm grateful my body works, but there's not an inch of it I like—wrong coloured skin, out of control hair, globules of fat everywhere, nails that crack and break. A face that will never be deemed pretty in a world where slim and pretty are the passports to happiness.

Yet sitting on the steps at the botanical gardens, I'm content. The warmth flowing through my body on the crisp autumn day is not just breastmilk—it's rightness. I'm married to the right man; I know this. I have the right children and I'm at home in my role as a mother. I feel it deep in my core. I'm acceptable as a mother but not as a woman. This, too, I feel deep in my core.

Even now, the image of this young woman with her three cherished babies is hard to reconcile with the middle-aged woman I've become and the six-foot-tall young men that replaced my babes-in-arms. To see myself at peace, knowing contentment and acceptance of my place in the world, is a stark reminder that everything passes. A transient world. A reminder that no matter how beautiful or ugly the moments, they will pass. The hopes, dreams, and expectations I held back then, have been and gone. Some fulfilled, some passed by. The hopes, dreams, and expectations I hold today will also pass by—some fulfilled and some passed by.

This precious image is wrapped around my heart. I still feel the warmth of Liam's body nestled into me and Hamish's soft caress, his body warm and snug in my arms.

BLESSED

I have three beautiful, healthy baby boys, my husband is permanently employed, I'm a trainee breastfeeding counsellor, and I've had virtually no musical work in the two years since we left Canberra. I'm once again caught between the juxtaposition of loving my role as wife, mother, friend, and counsellor, but desperately sad to have lost the career I'd always dreamed of. I decide to dig in, work hard, regain my skills, and get some work.

I find myself trying to practice the flute with one child at the breast, one sitting on the toilet calling for his bum to be wiped, and the other throwing a tantrum behind a door I'm holding closed with my foot. I decide practising by myself at home is too difficult, and in 2001, I enrol in a Graduate Diploma in Music at the Tasmanian Conservatorium—back to my university roots. But it's not the same. The heady days of making firm friendships and feeling a connected sense of community never arrive; I'm too old or too fat or have too many kids. I don't fit in.

I obtain the diploma and start applying for professional orchestral jobs. I spectacularly fail every single audition—the silent voice of my mother echoing through my head clear as crystal at every audition, "You're going to fail." And I fail every flute audition I ever attend.

I learn to sing instead.

I've barely left the house since Hamish was born and want something for myself, so I join a community choir. It's music and I figure a community choir will be a nice easing into the Tasmanian musical community. I haven't sung since leaving school, and exercising my musical skills in even a small capacity feels good. Seeing photos of myself performing does not; I'm at the peak of my weight gain. The fattest I've ever been. I decide I'll have to accept my weight and just relax into being a fat person and all that comes with it. A few weeks later, I see an ad for Weight Watchers; they're running a New Year's special offer and my short-lived acceptance of relaxing into being a fat person flies out the window along with a weekly Weight Watchers attendance fee.

Over the course of a year, I lose 34kg and win the 2003 Lifetime Member Award in the Weight Watchers Slimmer of the Year competition. I've done it purely by changing my diet and exercising more. A formula that's been around for as long as women have worried about weight. Except not for one single day did I manage to follow the *rules* of the Weight Watchers plan. I just managed to follow it sufficiently to lose weight. Mostly, I dropped into a binge-restrict cycle—something I was destined to become very good at in the years to come. My purging briefly rears its ugly head for a few weeks, but the associated misery just isn't worth it. Easier to starve. When I finally reach my "goal weight," for the first time in my life, I hear the words, "I'm so proud of you." I'm thirty-seven years old. I've gained and lost thirty or so kilos several times now, clinging to the wildly swinging pendulum of too much and too little.

My nervous joining of a community choir blossoms into private singing lessons and it's not long before I outgrow the choir and go in search of deeper waters. I only want to work with the best, so I audition for the Tasmanian Symphony Orchestra Chorus. I fail.

The Chorus Master chats to me and says I did a great job, but perhaps next time, *try not to be nervous*. It doesn't seem like very useful advice, but the fact that she mentions next time gives me the courage to give it one more go. This time I get in.

I spend eight years singing soprano in the chorus, accompanied by the Tasmanian Symphony Orchestra and doing a couple of interstate tours to Sydney and Adelaide. It's not how I dreamed of performing with the orchestra, but it's still really jolly satisfying. Fauré's *Requiem*. Handel's *Messiah*. Martin's *Mass for Double Choir*. Twice. And endless versions of *Zadok the Priest* and *Jerusalem*. I have a voice and I'm using it for something I love. I study singing a little harder and pass a few exams.

In 2003, as chance would have it, I bump into an old friend from my Ogilvie High School days and discover she's the musical director for an upcoming production of *Jesus Christ Superstar*.

"Do you want to play flute and piccolo in the band?" she asks.

Shit yeah!

I can't believe it. I'll be performing and meeting other musicians, doing shows, getting out of the house to do something unrelated to breastfeeding. I'll be performing music again. I can't wait!

I've arrived at the magical goal weight but still try to lose just a little bit more as a buffer zone. A more slender version of myself is more acceptable in the world of performance; I can't tell if it's real or imagined. I wear size eight clothes, sing in the TSO Chorus, and perform in *Jesus Christ Superstar*. Life feels blessed.

I practice like my life depends on it, turn up to the first rehearsal and remember once more why I pursue music my entire life. I love it. The deep sense of oneness and knowing in my belly. I can do this shit standing on my head. And I do. Not on my head—but seated in a chair in the pit at the Theatre Royal. The same theatre my father and uncle performed in on countless occasions decades ago. I spend ten years performing in musicals, revelling in the heady delights of rehearsals and sitzprobes, live audiences and musical camaraderie, a sense of competency, nights out socialising and drinking, bump-outs and after-parties. I'm paid to do what I love, and for just a moment, I forget I'm a middle-aged mum and reclaim some of the lost merriment of my university days.

It does wonders for my self-esteem but is not kind to our marriage. The sense of freedom I find in my musical life highlights a sense of regret I never knew I felt at home. Mick and I start to grow apart.

I'm offered a teaching job at a prestigious private girls' school. I meet a collection of gorgeous girls, all (most) excited to learn how to play the flute, and a team of instrumental teachers all passionate about the huge benefits music adds to education and working hard to create an enviable music department. I'm soon teaching not just groups but a growing number of private students where I get the opportunity to once again mentor young people—not just in the art of playing the flute, but teaching resilience, study techniques, passion, creativity, self-expression, confidence, working in groups or independently, and respect for the role we each play in life, wherever that may be. Many staff members come and go, but I stay and teach the flute there for thirteen years.

We finally have a sense of security in our Tasmanian lives. It was a rough start, but after six years in Hobart, both of us are working, our boys are happy and healthy, I adore my work, and at last I've found my community.

Kirsten returns to Hobart with her young family, and I'm thrilled to have a close friend nearby. I have enduring friendships with other beautiful people all over Australia, where time and distance make no difference. I tentatively make new friends in Hobart and stumble upon more variations of trust, understanding, resilience, and security in my friendships.

FOOD RULE 34

If I eat, I must exercise.

SAVING GRACE

I mother the three boys I birthed and the hundreds of girls I teach. I revel in flute and voice performance, while all the inevitable things that inevitably happen as our thirties pass by and fifties start staring at us in the mirror start to happen. I have an unsettled feeling in my belly.

In 2008, I obtain a Masters in Journalism, putting into practice my second favourite thing to do—write. But I'm hesitant to trust my writing ability, so I specialise in editing. The nitty-gritty of studying every word on a page and correcting the smallest of errors fits neatly into my perfectionist nature. I take on a voluntary role as a communications assistant, and three months later, I'm offered permanent part-time work. Between teaching, performing, singing, and being a communications assistant, I'm working long hours—too long. Something has to give, and after a public reprimand in my communications role for not using the appropriate chain of hierarchy to contact the institution CEO, I feel a familiar sense of utter humiliation and resign. I go back to what I know well—steering clear of large organisations and their inevitable politics.

Life with our boys is a busy mess of pride and joy as they win medals at soccer or awards in eisteddfods, and fear and despair when we're called yet again to the principal's office or the hospital. Our finances are limited but we're living in the age of helicopter parenting and over-scheduled children. We make the decision that they can play one sport each and learn one musical instrument each. With three kids, that's still a fair bit of taxiing around in my old Holden Commodore. Conor takes up gymnastics and the bassoon. Liam loves his soccer and reluctantly plays the clarinet. Hamish reluctantly plays soccer and learns to play the flute. Somewhere amongst all of that, Mick and I work and do all the normal things that normal families do. Conor commences high school and I've just got Liam and Hamish in primary school; the years are flying past fast. I collect the two younger boys from school one day and Liam promptly bursts into tears in the car. My little grade five boy who's all bravado on the outside and highly sensitive on the inside and reminds me so much of myself. He clings to a very strong set of moral values—that sometimes align with societal rules and sometimes do not. Sitting in the front seat, he angrily wipes away the tears and tells the tale.

"What's happened, Liam?"

"I told my teacher to get fucked."

"Liam!"

"Well, he told me to go and get the ball, but I wasn't the one who kicked it away and then the bell went, and he told me to go and get it anyway, and I told him the bell's gone and he has no control over me now, and he said he has control of me until 3:30 so I told him to get fucked and I left."

"Liam, we need to go back to the school and talk to the principal and sort things out. I'll drop Hamish home, then we'll go back."

I pull into the driveway at home and Liam hightails it out of the car before I can stop him and runs across the paddock down to nearby Boronia Beach. I panic. Mick says he'll come back when he's hungry. The school rings to give me their side of the story (not dissimilar to Liam's interpretation, except the teacher claims Liam kicked the ball away. In this circumstance, I believe Liam is correct). It takes forty-five minutes, but Liam comes back when he knows the school office is closed—and he's hungry. He receives two days of internal suspension. He never loses the anger at being wrongfully accused of kicking the ball away.

In April 2009, Mick and I take our three boys on our first ever proper holiday—a month in South-East Asia exploring the golden temples and hot sandy beaches in Thailand, the poverty of Phnom Phen, the ancient ruins of Angkor Wat, the traffic chaos, and the exquisite French pastries of Vietnam. We spend every penny scraped together over the course of a year, returning home with memories of tuk-tuks, beggars, mountains of marble, and push-starting a bus. We're in a big, happy, family-holiday bubble. By the end of the year, my slow unravelling begins.

I'm fat again. The momentary bubble of happiness from the Weight Watchers Slimmer of the Year competition lasts just three or four years before self-control starts waning, and binge eating starts taking over.

I'm ashamed of my inability to control food, yearning to be normal. Grandma pulls me aside for yet another chat about my weight problem— completely ignorant of the fact that I'm not ignorant about my weight. If there's one thing we fat people know, it's that we're fat. Food is my emotional panacea and life is full of emotion. My wardrobe is full of clothes from size eight to twenty-four.

Mick and I have been married for seventeen years. For the first twelve, I felt we were still in the honeymoon phase. That was five years ago. Now we've accrued a silent collection of unvoiced resentments and nearly two decades of familiarity bordering on contempt. We're mostly happy together, but cracks are starting to appear. Our communication strategies are slowly eroding.

I continue to bury myself in mothering and music—the two things in which I most strongly identify. But over time, both identities start to change and dwindle, my boys doing what all children do—growing up. And my career doing what many careers do—growing away. I become ever more fragile and ill-equipped for the onslaught of trials and tribulations that are about to test me.

Over the next few years, there are two more saving graces—two more people who make a world of difference in my life and complete my circle of twelve—my psychologist, and a new friend Sheree. Twelve amazing souls who stand by me when I least expect it—and least deserve it. Mick, The Girls (my sisters-at-heart from my conservatorium days), Sheree, Emma, Kerry, my psychologist, and three friends who make up my twelve pillars of strength in the trials to come.

I meet my psychologist in 2015 when I trudge along to my first appointment with no expectation that anything will change, *I'm beyond redemption,* my new mantra in life. As fate would have it, I'm truly blessed to accidentally stumble upon an angelic, patient, motherly soul, ready, willing, and able to take on the tangled mess I weave. Week by week, she patiently listens to my sorry tale, slowly teasing out the moments of my life I never even knew were a problem. Apparently, I have anxiety and depression and have always had them. *But that's my mother and sister, not me!*

I feel like Shrek's many-layered-onion, peeling back layer after layer of emotional protection swathed around me since childhood and so instinctive I no longer recognise the face behind the carefully constructed façade. It turns out, I don't know who I am.

THE LAMENTATIONS

I cry. I was never expressly taught—or told—that crying is a bad thing. Yet the message crept in anyway. Crying is a good thing—for other people. Crying is unacceptable—for me.

Over the course of six years, Mick and I lose ten family members—some younger, some older. Some close, some not so close. But the episodes of grief and stress escalate beyond my meagre capacity to cope, and the salty leakage from my eyeballs becomes commonplace. Decades of unacknowledged depression and anxiety bubble to the surface and the woman I've always been—the woman wrapped up tighter than an Egyptian mummy in layer upon layer of protective swaddling cloths—is slowly ripped apart, exposing a vulnerability I cannot comprehend and don't want to know about.

I sink into a lamentable abyss of maladaptive and ineffective coping behaviours, hidden away from all and sundry until hiding becomes impossible.

Slowly but surely, my relationships with everyone—my parents, my children, Mick, grandma, my friends, colleagues, students—are tipped on their head. A marriage I've chosen to stay in, despite all the shit we've put each other through, is now a relationship I'm terrified I'll lose—complacency and familiarity sinking in deep. While I cling to my default setting of doing all the things for all the people all the time, when all my metaphorical balls start falling out of the air, Mick is the one left holding them. He now does all the things for me all the time.

Resentments slip in for both of us. The fiercely independent, capable woman I've always been, is dependent and incapable. I hate it. I don't know who she is. I don't like her. As 2015 rolls into 2016, my identity evaporates.

LOSING MYSELF

I remember with absolute clarity the moment my first baby was placed in my arms. I was lying on the operating theatre table, having a caesarean I desperately didn't want, tearfully asking if all his fingers and toes were present and accounted for with little concern for more important body parts or physical conditions. The cord was cut, he was assessed, wrapped, and placed in my arms for Mick and I to adore while the surgeons did what they needed to do.

We cried with love and kissed each other and smothered our precious bundle in gentle kisses while inhaling the extraordinary scent of newborn baby. And we fell deeply in love—right there and then—with this miraculous new person. Until I held him in my arms, I didn't know there was a whole other way of loving. Not the passionate and lustful love of new romance. Or the eternal and fractious love of family. And not the gentle, patient, comfortable love of good friends. Holding my own baby in my arms for the first time burned an everlasting and unbreakable love into my heart and soul. The sights, sounds, and smells of my very own child, a physical part of myself, taught me there's nothing I wouldn't do to love, protect, and nurture my children—forever.

Those first hours, days, weeks, and months were filled with love and dependency, but I was raising this little person to leave me—raising an adult, not a child. Hopefully a strong, independent, resilient adult. Those early years—repeated with as much love and awe twice more as his younger brothers came into the world—flew by with frightening speed. Despite the moments I wished away (*This too shall pass!* too often chanted), they were the happiest years of my life. My very own little people—nursing at my breast, snuggling in my arms, crying for cuddles, and begging for independence. I never wanted to let them go.

Now I have young men instead. Strong, independent, resilient, talented, compassionate, extremely tall (well, two out of three), young men—making their own mistakes, creating their own communities, living their own lives. The early years of twenty-four-hour, seven days a week dependence on me has morphed into seeing them just two or three hours most weeks—on family dinner nights. The newborn babies I held in my arms and fell in love with have graduated from university, mastered the art of burger flipping and pizza delivery, broken the law and paid the consequences, fallen in love, fallen out of love, travelled, skied, survived music festivals, repaired carburettors, and held me when I broke. The light at the end of the tunnel, the one I focused on when overwhelmed by toddlers and teens, now burns so brightly I want to shield my eyes and stop the passage of time.

It's really hard to let go. We taught these young men how to read and write, clean toilets, and ride pushbikes. To cope with disappointments and humiliation, as well as success and pride. They've made mistakes—big and small—and made us proud more often than not. And every time they learned a new skill, they were just a little more independent and grown-up.

Motherhood is an overwhelming identity for me, one I can't and won't let go, but I find myself flailing about in unknown waters trying to discover what motherhood looks like when my children are adults. Watching them live lives I have no say in and hoping the choices they make now will be no worse than the choices Mick and I made when we too were young and full of dreams.

Adult conversations with young men I once potty trained are a surreal experience. Letting go is hard. Much harder than you might think when you're into yet another month of sleepless nights and cracked nipples—

when the years ahead are paved with the all-encompassing daily grind of school and sport, tears, and tantrums. Four years of my life spent as a passenger in my own car, supervising learner drivers and learning the true meaning of fear and powerlessness. Parenting brought me the happiest—and most exhausting—days of my life, and they're now behind me. I've lost my identity as a mother, my sense of self is crumbling away, and the broken woman left behind is not someone I recognise. I don't know how to be myself.

We hear about the importance of letting stuff go. Let emotions go. Let stress go. Let people go. Let your career/husband/kids/dog go. But it's not that easy, is it?

Many moons ago, I remember being at Questacon, The National Science & Technology Centre in Canberra. They have a free-fall slide which is basically a slippery dip where you hang from a bar and free-fall onto it. From the ground looking up, the drop is tiny; you free-fall a split second before you're on the slide and heading down. But hanging from the bar looking down, the drop is enormous. Despite knowing it's completely safe, biological instincts kick in to say what you're doing is unnatural; stop it right now. Your heart pounds, your breathing is rapid, and your body shakes. And the inside of your head screams, *I can't do it!* It's astonishingly difficult to override fear with logic and let go of that bar.

I cling to emotional issues and well-worn coping mechanisms with the same panicked grip. A biological instinct kicks in saying, *don't do it, don't do it*, and all the rational and logical statements in the world don't help. You know you have to do it, but overriding that instinctive fear mechanism is all-consuming and exhausting. Arachnophobes, aerophobes, and acrophobes all know exactly what I'm talking about. As do all the other phobes.

I seem to have multiple fears.

Fear of failure (atychiphobia). Fear of dogs (cynophobia). Fear of getting fat (pocrescophobia). They are my big three—and I've learned they all have proper scientific names which ironically makes me feel less alone. We all have fears; if you think you don't, you're wrong. But some are less obvious or intrusive than others. And some people have more extreme versions than others. My pocrescophobia is overwhelming. It rules my life and has escalated since 2012. If I can't overcome this fear, I will be trapped in eating disorder land forever.

It's a whirlwind of emotions—the celebrations and *hey, you look great!,* the assumptions that I'm now living this miraculously healthy life, a constant pressure on me to maintain thinness achieved through secret means, alternating periods of binging and starving, joining a gym and over exercising, honing all my eating disorder skills, and returning to purging. Whatever the goal weight is, it's unachievable. Because the goalposts always move. And if for some magical reason I were to feel comfortable at the goal, the stress of having to maintain the weight is somehow worse than losing it in the first place.

I have been fat. I have been thin. I was no less fearful when fat or thin. Losing the weight doesn't help the fear—at all. In fact, it makes it worse.

FOOD RULE 55

Only consume diet shakes.

HUG ME

There are three deaths: the first is when the body ceases to function.
The second is when the body is consigned to the grave.
The third is that moment, sometime in the future, when your name is spoken for the last time.

[David Eagleman]

I've never seen anyone die before my mother slips into a coma and the painful truth is, it's not a pretty sight. We often hear it's a privilege to be with someone at the end of their life and I find this to be true, but it's also distressing. I never expect to embark upon such a journey of grief, emotional trauma, and unravelling. It all begins with her cancer diagnosis.

Melbourne, February 2001. Hot days and muggy nights. The Olympic fever of Sydney 2000 has been and gone and the World Trade Centre Towers are still standing in New York City. I'm almost thirty-five years old and not fully cognisant of the fact that I'm living through the happiest and most satisfying years of my life, completely immersed in my protective cocoon of earth mother. My world is a blur of bedtime stories and rote learning times tables, and it's just six more months before I breastfeed for the last time. Hamish is turning two and we've jumped on the short flight across Bass Strait from Hobart to Melbourne to celebrate his birthday with my mother.

It's a trip we can't afford but it's less than a year since her breast cancer diagnosis and I'm conscious of the fragility of her life and scarcity of time. I want my children to know their grandmother, and her to know them, while she's here. She shows a devotion and affection to her grandchildren never evident with her own children. And this is the crux of why I'm in Melbourne sweltering through another stinking hot day; I'm fearful she'll die before I can ask the difficult questions.

"Why did you never hug me as a child?" I ask.

It's taken twenty-four hours to summon the courage to ask. Her husband is composing music in his studio and Hamish is having a cuddle on my lap.

"You didn't want to be hugged," she replies.

I'm momentarily speechless. What kind of child doesn't want to be hugged? Is the resentment I carried all these decades my fault?

"You were so independent," she adds.

She sits primly in her wicker chair with a mint-green turban disguising her chemotherapy-induced baldness.

"All of you were."

All of us. My mother delivered four healthy babies—losing Christian to SIDS—but my brother and sister weren't hugged either. I'd been too self-absorbed to notice this little titbit of information.

"You were all so difficult and misbehaved. Life gets stressful and busy with three children."

"I know that, mum. I have three kids and we hug them all the time. I can't imagine not hugging my children."

"Did you want to be hugged?" she asks.

It feels like she's laying the burden of my undemonstrative childhood at my feet.

"Don't all children want to be hugged?" I ask.

"Not always," she says.

It's the end of our conversation and we sit in silence, sipping earl grey tea in delicate china cups. Tea we've always prepared exactly the same way—strong with just a dash of milk. Two grown women with no capacity to engage in conflict, caught in an emotive discussion about a perceived failure of her mothering. I feel bad. It's a pointless question and there's no answer. She's dying and I've accused her of being a bad parent. For whatever reason, she was unable to hug her children, and there's no going back.

We never discuss it again, but she instigates a new hugging regime. I don't know if it's because she feels remorse for the lack of closeness to her children or if she's making a point about our conversation. Saying, *Look. I hug you. See?*

Whatever the reason, her hugs are foreign and unfamiliar. I feel uncomfortable with her affection. It's not how our relationship evolved. I learned affection and warmth from friends, my husband, and children—not my parents or grandparents. I was desperately independent as a child while simultaneously craving love and affection. I grew up feeling disconnected from everyone and unsure how to behave in the world. I came from a home that wasn't quite right but don't know how to heal the broken part of my soul—how to connect with the world and myself. It's another seventeen years before I start the healing process and recognise my childhood for what it was. Creative, colourful, inadequate, invalidating, neurotic, nomadic, unusual, unexpected. Like my grandmother before her, my mother did the best she knew how. It wasn't enough—but it was all she had to give.

My grandmother. In 2001, she's still a sprightly, energetic eighty-three years young. By the time my mother is terminally ill, grandma is ninety-one, and while she's blessed with good health and a fierce independence that runs in the women of our family, time stands still for no one. She becomes increasingly dependent on me for support. I feel an overwhelming sense of duty to care for the woman who cared so much for me as a child. Her demands are demanding and her demeanour demeaning. My weight is as fickle as the weather forecast—up and down with no predictable pattern. Running out of ideas and options after forty-three years, I decide to try diet shakes. It's fast and convenient. It lasts as long as all the other food rules. Less than a week.

I struggle with the emotional onslaught grandma subjects me to nearly every day. My hair is too long, too short. I should have let my children spend more time with her. I expected too much of her with my children. I don't appreciate anything enough. I should help her more. I should sit down and spend more time relaxing. I shouldn't be such a snob. I should never wear pink or red. I should be visiting her more often. I should be able to find the out-of-stock item at Woolworths—even though it's out of stock. I should be able to find shops that will cash cheques—even though nobody writes cheques anymore. I know she loves me; we often treat those we love the worst. But she never shows it. She doesn't do hugs either.

INTRODUCTION TO GRIEF

My mother and I never learn to connect emotionally, but over the nine years of her illness and eventual death, our relationship undergoes a slow metamorphosis. The vivacious, fussy, hypercritical, anxious, exasperating, independent woman I know—the woman who would wash clean clothes and clean dishes just to be sure they were clean—can no longer brush what's left of her hair or make her way unaided to the bathroom. She's utterly reliant on others for absolutely everything. I visit as much as possible to ease the burden on her aging husband and spend what time I can with her—unpacking boxes, doing housework, preparing food, running her bath, washing her hair.

In 2000, she's diagnosed with a stage four tumour in her breast. It's the size of a grapefruit, ready to burst through the skin, and during the mastectomy, cancerous lymph nodes are found and removed. The prognosis is poor, but she undergoes chemotherapy and radiation therapy, buying herself a very unexpected nine years—enough time to travel to all the places she's yearned to see and to meet every one of her six grandchildren.

The cancer spreads to her lungs and bones, leaving her hooked up to oxygen and in constant pain. She and her husband relocate to Hobart so she can be close to me and extended family. In February 2009, all their worldly possessions are packed up, and they buy a renovator's delight with a wild garden full of flowering gums and bright red geraniums, in a superb position around the corner from my house.

Everyone thinks she's mad to undergo such a stressful project, but I see the woman who has bequeathed me the stubborn determination to do whatever I set my mind to. She's quite literally deathly ill, with little time left, but she still takes on the task of a massive renovation. The house is completely gutted, and a new kitchen, bathroom, living areas, and bedrooms are built upstairs. Downstairs (aka The Dungeon) is an underground self-contained unit with a bedroom, kitchen, bathroom, living area, and practically no windows or natural light.

Many cups of tea are brewed and imbibed as plans are drawn up, colours and splashbacks chosen, and builders deconstruct and reconstruct above. They live in The Dungeon until May when my mother finally moves upstairs to the house of her dreams—generous windows spilling warm Tasmanian sunlight into the living areas and bringing gusts of clean, fresh air from the spectacular Derwent River views for her failing lungs.

We spend hours together, my mother directing while I carry out the unpacking of boxes, rearranging antique teapots, silverware, vintage dresses, and Russian dolls—all the things she's proudly collected from eBay over the years.

November 2009, I come into her new bedroom, with its polished floorboards and huge windows overlooking the leafy front yard with the giant magnolia tree, to see her sitting up in bed wearing bright red lipstick. Ambulance officers are on their way to the house again. And she probably won't go back to hospital—again.

She looks at me and says, "Do I look silly?"

I smile and say, "No. You look beautiful," and realise at that moment that our roles have completely reversed; I'm now parenting my mother.

Her demise plays on my mind; it's hard to watch. She's almost bed-bound and says she hopes not to last more than two months as she can't cope any more. I'm deeply conscious of what a sad life she's had, and despite laying the blame for my unhappy childhood largely at her feet, I feel nothing but compassion for this woman who is my mother.

Who suffered most of her life and is dying a painful, difficult death. I'm filled with regret for the times I was unkind, lacking empathy, and not understanding her more. I hope she will see Christmas. She hopes for only one thing, asking to see Vanessa one last time. It's an impossible task. Vanessa lives on the Gold Coast, and geographically the 2,500 kilometres is too great, my little sister too unstable and incapable of travelling on her own. I'm not even sure she's allowed to fly after the Australian Federal Police escorted her from the last plane she was on for fighting with a woman in the queue for the toilets. I'm distraught that I can't deliver the one thing my mother desires—to see her broken baby girl one last time.

The next day, she's in and out of a delirious state, looking me in the eye and asking, "Are you expecting a baby? Someone's expecting a baby."

Nobody we know is expecting a baby.

I don't know if it's the morphine playing tricks or if it's her failing body and cognitive functions, but I'm left with two dilemmas. Should I invite relatives to visit as soon as possible? Do they want to know she's dying? To come and see her? Will she even recognise them by next week? Maybe she'll be completely lucid. Maybe not. How can I know?

And then, how much do I involve my children? They're early teens now and I don't know whether to let them witness her decline or if they should be there at the end if possible. There are no guidelines or precedents for me in this situation; I'm out of my depth. Everyone looks to me for guidance, but I don't know what to do. I ring carers, family, and friends, and organise everything. I do all the things for all the people all the time. It's my default setting and the way I can most effectively distance myself from all emotions.

At 10:35 a.m. on Friday, 13 November 2009, my mother dies. She's sixty-five years old. Despite the knowing and the waiting, her death is a shock.

Wednesday, she's in great spirits, energetic, bossing everyone around. Thursday, she wakes with the worst pain she's ever experienced, and palliative care suggests taking more frequent doses of morphine. I spend all day with her, then come back in the evening to help her husband move her into a more comfortable position. As we manoeuvre her down the bed beneath the pale blue floral Laura Ashley quilt, her eyes pop open and she looks at me and smiles. She's always had a most beautiful smile. She slips into a coma that night.

Friday morning, I take Mick and the boys over before my ninety-one-year-old grandmother arrives saying, "It's okay, mum's here. Your mother is here." I can't stop crying, ashamed of my weakness. Tears aren't shed in our family.

My mother's breathing is increasingly ragged while the boys are busy moving the grand piano, baking a cake, rearranging furniture. The day is glorious, still and sunny, and the garden in full bloom. The air is filled with the sounds of cockatoos and rosellas and the Derwent River splashing on the nearby rocks. We all spend time with her, saying goodbye, kissing her forehead.

I spend the morning in bed with her, holding her hand, saying I'm sorry for everything I ever did wrong and that I love her. I barely leave her side, trying to compress a lifetime of lost connection into the last hours of her life. I'm crying and squeezing her hand while watching her face contorted into a permanent mask of fear and pain. Her eyes pop open for a moment and she looks deeply distressed, but then gradually relaxes, her pulse slowing, and eventually her breathing stops. Her fingers, dark purple due to lack of circulation for as long as I can remember, become white. I can't believe my mother's gone.

I ring Vanessa to let her know our mother is dead. She sobs down the phone, then starts screaming at the people in her living room to get out because her mother has just died. We talk on the phone for quite a while, then she says, "I love you." I phone my brother and sob, and he tries to comfort me. I phone dad, and we both cry. I can't do any more phone calls and pass the job onto Mick.

After the calls are made, my mother's husband sits down, and we have a cup of tea. He reads out messages she left in a palliative care kit. She leaves kind words for a small number of people. For me, it's very simple, "Thank you for your friendship, Simone."

Somehow, my heart cracks with the message. I know how deeply heartfelt it is from my mother; it's the kindest thing she's ever said to me. And I'm broken-hearted for her own struggle to give and receive love. For all my demonising of her faults, at the heart of it, my mother was a deeply sensitive, anxious, compassionate, and broken woman.

The following days pass in a flurry of activity, and with my mother gone, the primary person to care for is her husband—a man in his seventies who's now buried two wives with breast cancer. There's no time to grieve; there are arrangements to be made. So, I get busy and make arrangements.

Grandma has lost her only daughter. I'm deeply conscious that there's no good age to lose a child, and her grief must be overwhelming. I can't imagine how it feels, but she shows no emotion and sheds no tears. She's not one for grieving or funerals but remembers in her own way—planting a magnolia tree my mother gave her and creating little memorials of photos and knick-knacks all over her house. Both my mother and grandmother had a deep and abiding love for literature, so when grandma chooses a poem that she wants to be read at the funeral, I don't hesitate.

> *Do not stand at my grave and weep*
> *I am not there, I do not sleep*
> *I am a thousand winds that blow*
> *I am the diamond glint on snow*
> *I am the sunlight on ripened grain*
> *I am the gentle, gentle autumn rain*
> *Do not stand at my grave and weep*
> *I am not there, I do not sleep*
> *When you awake in the morning hush*
> *I am the swift uplifting rush*
> *Of quiet birds in circling flight*
> *I am the soft, soft starlight, starlight at night*
> *Do not stand at my grave and weep*
> *I am not there, I do not sleep*
> *[Elizabeth Frye]*

FOOD RULE 89

If I eat, I purge.

AN ACT OF DESPERATION

I barely have time to grieve for my mother. Life demands what it demands, and work, children, family, and commitments all come rolling back in. So does grandma. Now that my mother is unable to care for her, I pick up the reins and do my best to be a dutiful granddaughter. She vacillates between calling me a roaring success with my incredible musical abilities (which she's rarely seen in action) and a snobby, fat, woman who should never wear the colours pink or red and needs regular reminders that, "You're far from perfect you know." Days are busy and the months turn into years.

By February 2012, I'm forty-six years old and desperate. Despite eating less and walking more, my weight's going up—a fact grandma never fails to remind me. I'm miserable and I'm pissed off. With tear-stained reluctance, I sign up for a gym membership.

I meet the owner, Sheree, when I'm once again fat and desperate, all my previous exercise efforts now no longer able to keep menopause and overeating at bay. At first, she's my gym instructor, but I'm instinctively drawn to her honesty and empathy, and we eventually become firm friends. The older you get, the harder it is to find new friends—it feels like a lot of effort for the potential risk of being emotionally shattered. But with Sheree, not only do we get on well, but she provides a listening ear and a shoulder to cry on, and her shoulders are strong enough to bear my burdens without distress, held up by her deep and abiding faith in God, which is something I know nothing about. She is—in so many ways—completely different from all my previous friendships.

Exercising regularly changes my life—toning my body, turning fat to muscle, allowing me to enjoy the great outdoors, giving me a safe place to socialise daily, and saving my sanity in more ways than I can possibly count. I honestly don't know where I would be any more without regular exercise. I decide any food consumption can be tolerated if I compensate with exercise.

Two decades earlier, I swore to never return to a gym. They're isolationist, judgmental, sweaty places, where no normal human ever finds pleasure. Full of competitive Lycra-clad skinny girls and leering, bicep-flexing muscle boys, where narcissism trumps nurture. That's my experience of gyms. I traipse up the stairs to the newly opened women-only gym. Within minutes of telling my sorry tale, we're both in tears.

"You need strength training," declares Sheree with passion and optimism. "Get strong—in body, mind, and spirit."

I turn up the next day and fall in love. Not with exercise—that comes later—but with the people. The primary clientele are middle-aged women of every shape, size, athletic ability, and socioeconomic status. They're just like me. They wear normal clothes—no Lycra in sight—and are kind, empathetic, and understanding. Sheree and her team know every member, create a community, and focus on building strength, health, flexibility, and longevity—not caring who's the thinnest, prettiest, strongest, or fittest. It takes a village to raise a child but a community to support our eternal inner child. I'm nurtured.

By April, the daily trek to stand upon my scales shows nothing has budged. I've battled weight my entire life and I'm exhausted. I'm fat and getting fatter. I'm performing on stage with Conor in a touring production of Bizet's *Carmen*. The dress fittings are humiliating and I'm conscious of the many eyes that will peer down my ample bosom, exposed by the corsets we're ensconced in beneath our colourful peasant dresses. In tears and desperation, I meet with an obesity surgeon. It's Thursday; he has a cancellation Monday. I book in, have a lap band wrapped around the opening to my stomach, and change my life.

The adjustable gastric band, now securely attached to my insides and connected to a port that I can feel through my belly, is like an inflatable silicone donut where the surgeon increases and decreases the fluid in the band to make the opening to the stomach larger or smaller—therefore restricting food intake. It seems like a good idea. It takes me no time at all to turn it into surgical bulimia.

Ashamed at having to resort to such drastic measures, I tell only The Girls, Mick, and Sheree at the gym. Nobody thinks it's a good idea, but I know they'll never understand the deep-rooted disgust in myself that I feel every moment of the day. Mick supports my wish to be more comfortable in myself, while simultaneously feeling mystified as to why what I have isn't enough. He is aware of my body horror, but unaware how deep-rooted and linked to my sense of self my physical body has become.

I turn up to *Carmen* rehearsals five days after the laparoscopic surgery, telling nobody about the five little cuts in my belly and my new requirement to live on liquids for a month. The director decides I'm the perfect person to stand on a table in the bar scene, ending with a fist-pumping salute. I valiantly climb up and down from the table in rehearsals, punching my arm high in the air while singing in full voice with a well-supported diaphragm and not letting anyone know of my recent surgery—not even my son. My head spins and my belly hurts but the fist pump feels like the first success I've experienced in a long time.

At first, I love the lap band; I don't care what other people think. I'm never hungry and I'm losing weight. Soon, I figure out how to purge with ease. It's not deliberate; I accidentally eat sushi too fast, blocking the opening of the stomach so no food can go down at all. The ensuing pain is so overwhelming, I purge. I haven't purged for years, but with a lap band, it's so easy. The food, just sitting on top of the stomach, quickly fills up the oesophagus until there is no option but to purge. By the end of the year, I'm purging dozens of times per day. I don't mention this to the surgeon, and he never asks. Mick never notices.

The trouble with lap bands—if you haven't spent much time thinking about it—is that healthy foods are harder to consume than unhealthy foods. Chocolate and ice cream slides down easily. Smoothies and milkshakes can be consumed in large quantities with no immediate consequence. But tiny bowls of salad or chicken drumsticks are incredibly difficult to keep down. Grandma approves of my weight loss—at any cost. I visit her most days, and the incessant comments on my weight and appearance become dotted with positive observations.

Like all the other weight loss endeavours I embarked on in the past, I fail to follow the rules of the lap band. I get tired of fluids before the fluids phase is over. Tired of mushy stuff before the mushy phase is over. I don't lie to my surgeon but strategically omit key facts such as the number of times I vomit per day, the speed at which I cannot stop myself eating, and the water I wash all my meals down with despite being told not to consume liquids with meals. But just like my time at Weight Watchers, I lose the weight and look like a big success despite breaking the rules every single day.

Constant compliments on my slimmed-down body fuel the desire to maintain my successful weight loss strategy. Within a couple of years, vomiting is not just a daily affair, it's escalated to most meals and purging up to thirty times a day. By now, Mick has started to notice but is unaware of the intensity and frequency. I convince him it's just lap band related, and he believes me, content to live in his little bubble of, "She'll tell me when she's ready." My children are teenagers; they barely notice me. Despite never having had much care or respect for my body, I don't want to be put in a position where the lap band has to be removed. When I start vomiting bile, I get a fright. It tastes disgusting and I've kept almost no food or drink down for nearly a week. I go through periods of reflux so intense even hospital staff can't ease it when I'm admitted. Each time, I'm instructed to rest the band with just fluids for a few days and to have the band loosened so I can eat more easily. After a while, I always get it tightened again. When I can no longer swallow water without vomiting, an x-ray reveals that my stomach has herniated above the build-up of scar tissue beneath the band. The band is replaced. I make the assumption that it's due to excessive vomiting, but I don't ask and nobody tells me. I now have a love-hate relationship with the band. I love that it stops me eating properly. I hate that I can't eat properly. Vomiting is exhausting, and food tastes like failure.

I don't savour beautiful textures and flavours. I never mindfully and sensuously nibble delicacies, inhale aromas, and luxuriate in the tantalising sensations on my tastebuds. When I eat, I scoff food down like a starving woman fighting a horde of ravenous dogs, scratching around for the last morsel on a carcass. Washed down with guilt and loathing and fear, and an overwhelming sense of failure, I've done it again. I've eaten food I didn't want, in a manner I didn't like. I've failed myself.

But the food in my fridge sings to me—really sings. All day long, I think about food. *What am I going to eat, should I eat it, can I grab that and hide away with it, can I sneak a few of those and nobody will notice, how many calories are in that, can I skip a day of eating, can I fit any more in, if I eat fast enough can I throw it up, how many days can I go without food, will anyone notice if I have another one, what shall I eat when I go home, is there any cheesecake left, how long since I last ate, can I eat yet?* It never stops. The dialogue is incessant—all . . . the . . . time.

If I manage to distract myself long enough to do something else for a short period of time, when I glance up, walk past the kitchen on the way to the bathroom, hear someone open the fridge, or smell something cooking, the gentle siren song of the food in my fridge starts up.

It's a delicate melody with a very soft pulse—no time signature, no regularity. Just gentle melodic fluctuations and close harmonies slithering their way into my soul. It starts quietly, inaudibly, but before I know it, I'm hypnotised by the call of the cheese and the toast, the yoghurt and the chocolate. The calls get louder and more incessant, stronger and more powerful, until I can no longer resist. I'm drawn to the fridge, the door opens, and the food is chanting, *Eat me! Eat me!* I'm Alice down the rabbit hole—bewildered by the world around me and the food I'm consuming.

It tastes like failure. Day in and day out, I eat failure, or I don't eat at all. And that failure is an emotion so powerful it's almost tangible; I could reach out and touch it. Food tastes like failure and failure is a feeling—characterised by shame, anger, and being overwhelmed. Which, according to the feelings wheel, translates to sad, mad, and scared. I live my life sad, mad, and scared. Or, in clinical terms, anxious and depressed.

Another belief is etched deep into my soul. Feelings are facts. When I feel like a failure—when I'm ashamed and angry at myself and overwhelmed with the sense of inevitability of my own stupidity—these become the facts. Not only do I feel stupid, I AM stupid. Not only do I feel fat, I AM fat. I'm fat and old and ugly and despised by others for my weakness and self-absorption. When I eat, I feel these things, and they feel like facts.

These factual feelings consume me. When external stressors escalate, a desperate desire to numb myself into oblivion with my medley of maladaptive behaviours takes over. My lap band stitches are barely healed before Vanessa's mental health issues begin to roar to an ugly climax.

LITTLE SISTER

I believe in angels. I always have and always will. My first—and forever—angel is my baby brother Christian. Despite grandma declaring I can't believe in angels if I don't believe in God, I believe anyway. There are no rules when it comes to faith; I can believe what I want.

On 04 July 2012, my sister joins Christian to watch over me, cleansed of all her mortal imperfections.

In 1997, she's twenty-six years old, studying drama with a friend, and drinks whiskey for the first time. She's barely drunk alcohol before. Within six weeks, she's an alcoholic. Fourteen years later, she's dead.

In May 2012, my twenty-four-year-old nephew rings to say Vanessa's in hospital, really ill with alcohol-related liver failure but non-compliant and trying to escape. They admit her for two nights under a Guardianship Clause, give blood transfusions, antibiotics, potassium, and fluids, attempting to drain abdominal fluid build-up. No pain relief is given as they don't want to strain her already damaged liver. Despite a high tolerance for pain, she can't stand the procedure and only 300ml is drained before she begs them to stop. Two days of treatment is enough for her to regain the strength to get up and run away from the hospital, still in her pyjamas, with three cannulas attached. She pulls them out at home and bleeds everywhere.

I make the four-hour flight to the Gold Coast to spend time with her and set up support services for Vanessa and Jamie. After years of rarely talking, we get to know each other again. She greets me at the door—warm, welcoming, and her funny bubbly self. I think things will be okay. I can see her big swollen tummy, her tiny frame looking seven months pregnant. She's named the swollen belly, Baby Eliza. She's bleeding internally and can barely walk with the pain. She's jaundiced and puffy but still my little sister with her shiny jet-black hair below her waist. She lives in pyjamas, woolly coats, and a pink beanie with a woollen tassel. She's always cold, despite living in Australia's famous Gold Coast, with its surf beaches and sunshine.

I'm mentally prepared for how she looks and behaves, but not prepared for the squalid conditions she lives in. Once so fastidiously clean and tidy that no coffee cup touched the coffee table, she now lives in filth. Jamie, now living with a group of friends and unable to manage her erratic behaviour and decrepit living conditions, doesn't know how to look after her; he's too young and he's never grown up with normality.

Two cats go to the toilet anywhere they like. Years of smoking without cleaning has left walls stained mustard yellow. The kitchen and bathroom are feral with caked-on grease and dust, and the once-cream stair banister is now dark brown. My first night is spent in a huge bed with a blood-stained sheet, hideously stained pillows, a child-size doona, and an old woollen blanket covered in grease. I wear as many layers of clothing as I can find, use the doona as a sheet, a towel over the pillows, and manage a full three hours of sleep. The next day, I add $600 to our credit card debt for food, cleaning products, linen, and absent necessities like pegs, light globes, and toilet paper. I dedicate two days to scrubbing everything I set eyes on.

Vanessa has haemorrhoids and one is huge, engorged, and bleeding. She thinks nobody believes how bad it is and coerces me into looking at her bum. A haemorrhoid the size of a lemon momentarily pops out of her arse, like a turtle looking at the view. I promptly buy her a haemorrhoid pillow.

Random bruises appear, and her eyesight deteriorates. She's exhausted and sleeping all the time. My role is to set up support services so she won't be alone and floundering, and Jamie feels supported. It's a monumental task.

I obtain hospital records so her primary care physician can write referrals for home assistance. He's the most uncompassionate human I've ever had the displeasure to meet. He doesn't look at or speak to Vanessa. Doesn't examine her or show any care but keeps repeating she must return to hospital. I look him in the eye and ask directly, "Is she going to die?" He smiles and shrugs his shoulders, refusing to write referrals for home assistance, and we leave in disgust.

Dad's about to undergo major heart surgery in Hobart and my looming performances for *Carmen* require me to return home. I attend an AL-ANON meeting before I leave, sobbing throughout my sharing, and I'm desperate for advice on Gold Coast services that anyone can share after the meeting. I frantically follow up recommendations and discover a palliative care nursing service. I email them Vanessa's medical records that discuss low platelets, low haemoglobin, enlarged liver, internal bleeding, ascites and varices, and other things I don't understand. I add my personal (wholly uneducated) appraisal of my forty-year-old sister:

- swollen belly
- abdominal pain
- jaundiced
- constant diarrhoea—black tarry stools
- blood seeping from lower lip
- bleeding from haemorrhoid
- nausea
- vomiting
- swollen feet
- weak
- faint
- sleeping more and more
- no appetite
- not eating
- drinking a little water, sip of orange juice, small amount of whiskey
- still smoking

She sleeps on a mattress on the garage floor, because she's too weak to climb stairs. She's incontinent, in pain, and doesn't have the strength to lift her body weight. I've seen animals treated with more dignity.

I barely eat—the lap band has only been in about six weeks.

The palliative care nurses are amazing and put me in touch with a doctor who visits Vanessa at her home. He patiently explains the reality of her declining health, then asks if she's aware that by staying home and refusing medical treatment, she will die. She says yes. He talks to us both at length, then agrees to sign her up as a palliative patient. We're given immediate access to angelic nurses and amazing social workers, and receive a wheelchair, hospital bed, commode, and portable shower for downstairs in her tiny flat. She's finally being treated with dignity, and I reluctantly head back home to musical and family commitments, hoping like hell that I get to see her again. Jamie is left in charge of caring for his dying mother.

Dad's in intensive care looking pale and grey, but the multiple bypass surgery has gone well and he recovers remarkably quickly for a seventy-nine-year-old. The nursing staff advise me not to let him know just yet that his youngest child is dying.

STALKED BY DEMONS

The return to ordinary life is not ordinary. The daily trek to grandma is soul-destroying.

Conor's unexpectedly skipped year eleven and started university a year early. Liam is redefining the definition of teenage rebellion. Hamish has morphed into surly adolescence. Mick feels abandoned. I reschedule all the missed teaching and performances from my time away. Days pass by in a flurry of busyness, and moments of sanity have fled to the distant past. I'm not coping, and my innate sense of self-destruction rises to the surface.

The toilet bowl is filthy. The once pristine porcelain is now stained with caked-on shit, the water a murky swirl of rust and unflushed paper. Crumbs of filth are speckled around the rim—the origins of which don't bear thinking. If I had an ounce of dignity, I'd exit the cubicle before getting any closer. Instead, my dignity has fled, along with the toilet brush and disinfectant apparently.

There are eight cubicles in the shopping centre bathrooms and this one is furthest from the door. With a little luck, nobody will notice my feet facing the wrong way, or hear me gagging and retching as the last shreds of lunch are barfed into the bowl.

After I've purged, I'll have a ludicrous desire to feed the hole in my belly—which is one hundred per cent emotional and zero per cent hunger.

I'm pointlessly trying to fill a hole in my starving soul while mindlessly feeding a tiredness that won't go away with a few fast carbs. The emotional strain of recent months flushed away with the rest of the crap in the bowl.

The ritual is over. I press the button and hope like hell it flushes the evidence away, then emerge to wash my hands, glancing into the mirror to discover the toilet is not the only thing I flushed; my face is a red and splotchy mess. The tears are impossible to stop when your fingers are down your throat. This isn't how a grown woman is meant to behave; it's the very definition of undignified.

I'm a grown woman who's slimming down with the aid of the lap band and I need new clothes. It's winter in Hobart. Swimsuits are on sale because nobody in their right mind buys a swimsuit in a Tasmanian winter—the waters of the Derwent River flowing straight from Hobart to Antarctica with little land in between. I'm never quite sure what size clothing I should be in; I've been most of the sizes that exist. I grab a size sixteen, a suck-all-your-flabby-bits-in black tankini, and head to the change rooms to try it on. I strip down to my knickers and pull the top over my head.

I'm stuck, my G cup boobs squished halfway to my belly, arms sticking out at awkward angles. I can see myself in the mirror looking like a deformed tree of flesh, unable to do anything but sway in the wind. I start to panic, huffing and puffing in the change rooms, desperate to extract myself from a size sixteen I clearly do not fit into. I don't care if I tear the tankini into tiny little pieces; I just need to escape and get out of the department store. After several minutes of *ahs* and *huffs* and *oohs* and deep breaths, I finally free my naked torso from the Lycra death trap. It sounds like I've been having an orgasm in the change room for the past five minutes. I whip my own clothes back on, stuff the swimsuit onto the hangers, and exit the little cubicle, avoiding all eye contact with staff and customers. I decide I don't need a winter swimsuit.

GUARDED BY ANGELS

A few more weeks go by, and Jamie calls to say the doctor has never seen anyone with such a low haemoglobin level. Without a transfusion, my sister will soon die. Her haemoglobin is 4g/dl. I visit grandma to tell her Vanessa is not just sick, she's dying. She takes a deep breath and sighs, gives me photos and trinkets to take back, and sends her love. I don't tell dad. I fly back to the Gold Coast.

She's deteriorated rapidly—more grey than yellow and barely walking. Most people in her condition wouldn't walk at all, but there's a will of iron that runs through the women in our family. Jamie and I support her on either side as she slowly shuffles from lounge to bed, but after a few steps, her legs give out and we drag her.

The first night back, I go to bed around 2:15 a.m. She calls out at 3:30 a.m. (my entire sleep for the evening) needing help to get to the toilet. I optimistically think I can do this; she's tiny and there's nothing left of her. We shuffle about six steps before her legs give out and I drag her the rest of the way, grateful not only for the strength I've gained from the gym but knowing how to switch on my core, use my legs, and protect my dodgy back. Vanessa's on the floor in front of the toilet, so I hoist her up onto the seat. Her pink beanie falls in, and she still has her pants on. We burst out laughing, then spend several minutes wiggling them off. I beg and beg and beg her to let me set her up permanently in the living room—with the hospital bed, television, and commode. She refuses point blank; it won't look right.

The next day, she has a burst of energy. I'm standing in the kitchen holding a tea towel when *Party Rock Anthem* starts playing on the television. She gets out of her chair, cigarette in hand, wearing pj's, slippers, a purple woolly jacket, and a pink beanie, and starts shuffling—a dance trend I've heard of but have no idea how to execute. She's ecstatic that she can still shake it and has a cheeky grin on her face. It's the last time I ever see her happy.

On the second night, she calls out at 1:45 a.m. This time, she's tried to get to the toilet by herself, fallen, and cracked her head on the ground. She has a huge egg on the back of her head, and there's a small pool of blood on the floor. I manoeuvre her to the bathroom and mop up the blood.

Vanessa finally relents, and we set up the lounge room with the hospital bed, her two mangy cats sleeping at her feet. I learn to empty commodes, draw up syringes, and inject morphine into a butterfly clip. My heart is filled with sorrow when I see my twenty-four-year-old nephew effortlessly carry his mother to bed.

She can no longer hold her glass of whiskey or light her own cigarette but always has them at arms' length. We start doing shifts sitting with her. Jamie stays by her side while I sleep until 2 a.m., then I sit with her until morning. She can't sit up without assistance, constantly trembles, breathes rapidly, and has a really fast heartbeat. She sleeps most of the time but occasionally wakes and tries to joke with the constant visitors. She apologises endlessly that she isn't much fun and can't get anyone a cup of tea or a biscuit. Her favourite Foxtel shows play constantly in the background, the theme song to *Prisoner* serenading us day in and day out.

She's only awake for short periods of time, but we spend every one of her waking minutes talking about life and death and all the things that have happened. I record videos for dad and grandma. She asks me to look out for Jamie once she's gone.

Word gets out that she hasn't got long left. I want to steal a Visiting Hours sign to slow the endless stream of crying visitors from the complex she lives in—holding her hand, telling her what a big heart she has, what a good friend she is, and how much everyone loves her.

A definition of *not fun* is phoning your father to say his daughter isn't just sick, she's dying and close to the end. He's so happy to be just home from hospital and healing so well from the bypass surgery. I tell him the news. They speak at length then say goodbye. Dad never talks to his youngest child again, but their estrangement has ended, and great love is declared all around. He's sobbing, and my heart breaks for him.

On Thursday, I ask one of Vanessa's least loopy friends to sit with her so I can take Jamie out for dinner. We both need a break from the twenty-four-hour nursing routine, and we're gone no more than two hours. When we return, four of her friends are watching television, drinking her wine, and eating her food. They say she started snoring weirdly about an hour ago. I look at them like they're idiots and tell them she's most likely in a coma and can't breathe properly. I've seen my mother in a coma and the similarities are frightening. I lower the head of the bed so her airway is a bit clearer and her breathing eases. I send them all away. I phone the palliative care nurses and describe what's going on; they confirm that she's most likely in a coma. A nurse comes over later on. Vanessa said earlier in the day she would die tonight; she likes to get her own way but makes it through the night.

There's a little guardian angel I bought for her pinned to the top of her pyjamas.

As you go off on your journey to see the world anew,
This little angel is given to take special care of you.
So keep her with you always, tucked in a secret place,
She'll be your guardian angel and always keep you safe.

Vanessa is in a coma for twenty-two hours before leaving this earthly plane at 6 p.m. on Friday, 04 July 2012.

Her body is donated to science.

My sister. Beautiful. Funny. Damaged. Depressed. Loving. Supportive. Exotic. Anxious. Sensitive. Stubborn. Caring. Independent. Gone.

FOOD RULE 144

If I eat, I self-harm.

GRANDPA MAURICE

It takes just a few short days to organise Vanessa's funeral. I book a golf club. She hated golf, but the grounds are so pretty, overlooking an artificial lake with lilypads and ducks. It's very reasonably priced. Mick and I are not as poor as we once were—and certainly a lot wealthier than Vanessa and her son—but eight weeks of caring for and supporting Vanessa, and cancelling all my students while away, has taken a financial toll on our meagre income, and we're skint. I ask dad and grandma to fund the funeral (technically a wake, as her body lies with the Queensland Body Bequest programme). $400 does us nicely.

I write a eulogy for the third time in three years; I'm getting good at them now—my father-in-law, my mother, and my little sister. I read out *Do Not Stand at My Grave and Weep* again, then fly home via Canberra to meet Mick at his mum's house. His dad passed away in 2008 after a long battle with emphysema. Now not only is his mum's health deteriorating but it's abundantly clear her dementia is getting pretty bad. I look into her eyes and see the lights going out, listening to the same conversation so frequently it's like *Groundhog Day*. As we leave her house, we're not sure we'll ever see her again. Mick is sobbing.

We fly back to Hobart for a night then jump in the car for a four-hour drive and a mid-winter stay at the world heritage Cradle Mountain National Park in Tasmania's central highlands. It's Mick's fiftieth birthday and we've barely seen each other in three months. Serendipitously, I'd organised the surprise trip to the luxury King Billy suite at the very comfortable Cradle Mountain Lodge, long before I spent all our money on toilet paper and disinfectant at Vanessa's house.

We're barely out of Hobart before I get a call from my cousin.

"Hi, Simone. I'm sorry to hear about your sister and sorry to ring you with this news so soon after, but Grandpa Maurice died last night."

I hate phone calls.

I start tallying the deaths from the past three years—Mick's dad, my mother, Mick's aunt, my cousin, another of Mick's aunts, my sister, my grandfather. Sure, most of them are old and led good lives, but I feel it would be kind of nice to get a year off. My grandfather leaves instructions that there's to be no funeral so there's no eulogy to write and no opportunity to say goodbye. I have no idea where his ashes are scattered.

Grandma married Maurice Conley in 1941. They were the love story of southern Tasmania's Bruny Island, and until his dying day, Grandpa Maurice could recall seeing her stepping off the ferry for the first time. *She was a bit of alright.* Their marriage lasted a tumultuous thirty-five years of drunken, adulterous turmoil before grandma walked out and moved to Queensland's sunny Gold Coast to live with my parents in our toy shop, just as my young brother and sister were born.

I interviewed my grandfather a few years before he died, trying to understand why he became an alcoholic and a philanderer—both of which he denied. I found no answer but learned of the many hardships he was emotionally ill-equipped to deal with that contributed to a difficult life. I could see the will of iron, fierce intellect and emotional fragility that resurfaces in my own children three generations later. Growing up on the rural bush haven that is Bruny Island during the depression, his parents and their seven sons lost almost everything and were very poor. He left school at thirteen to work in the family sawmill, and at fifteen started a job driving steam logging locomotives.

"That's why my back's like it is today. I got caught up in the timing shaft. Completely stripped off all my winter gear from end to end in two seconds. The timing coupling just caught, and then all my winter clothes, my flannel underpants, completely stripped and took the socks out of my boots. Everything was gone. All I had left on was the tape off a singlet 'round my neck. My back's like a shelly beach where the coupling went up and down and ground in my back and all my hip. There was a bloke there and an old motorbike. He drove me home to get some more clothes. It was half-past four in the afternoon, [the boss] said, 'When he goes home to get clothes on, he better have the rest of the afternoon off.' If it could have spun me, I would have been mincemeat, but it couldn't spin me because of the wood box."

As painful as the accident must have been, emotional scarring happened in a car accident where he inadvertently killed a young couple on their motorcycle as they unexpectedly came hurtling out of the native bushland onto the narrow gravel road. Shortly after that, he left Bruny and took up a position as a prison guard at Hobart's Risdon Prison. My grandmother never spoke a kind word about that job, and the family always remembered Maurice as a ladies' man and a heavy drinker after that. A man who drank vodka at work and threw away his marriage with affairs. A man who was argumentative and foolish when on a drinking binge and easily seduced by women all his life.

Another accident years later left Maurice with a broken neck. Living back on Bruny in 1970—after his marriage ended and an electrical fire burned down his block of units in Hobart—Maurice tripped in long grass, fell over a retaining wall, and crashed headfirst into a concrete verandah. The first medical help came from the local nurse who inexplicably dragged him around for hours attempting to make him walk. He was airlifted to the Austin Hospital in Melbourne for intensive treatment. Maurice was unable to move anything but his tongue for the first few months.

"So, you'd have to think of nothing. We had a pegboard ceiling—a huge, big pegboard ceiling. So, I'd count the holes in the pegboard ceiling: corner-to-corner, crossways, and every way. Interesting life that was, 'cause you couldn't move. Just look up."

Maurice was never expected to walk again. When he finally recovered, he told the doctors, "This is a miracle. You cured me," but they simply said, "We done nothing for you. We don't know how; you should never come outa' that."

Recovering from a broken spine wasn't the first miracle Maurice believed happened to him. His family were Catholics considered religious hypocrites in the community.

"I know the time when my grandfather was dying, and the good Catholics were down there, and they thought he had hours to live so [the priest] came straight to the house and came in to do the Last Rites. He come to out of his unconsciousness and said, 'Get that bastard out of this bloody house,' and he lived another twenty years. So, the priest cured him."

Maurice also remembers a much-cherished aunt sent home to die after a cart accident, who cured herself through faith in Christian Science and lived another forty years. But his own faith was shattered when he and grandma took in a four-year-old child who died from stomach cancer three months later.

"Her name was Lisa, and while there she was like a little angel. She got cancer and died the most terrible agonising death that I ever seen. Standing up in hospital screaming in intense pain, and I switched back to Christian Science in desperation—the last hope. I stood back and watched, and it didn't work, and I lost all faith. Everybody at the last looks for something that probably doesn't exist. You'd only do it in desperation."

I hear Lisa's story repeatedly throughout my life. My mother was a young child when Lisa died and remembers her well; my middle name is Lisa as a tribute to her. Maurice's loss of faith also played a part in my own life when both my grandparents became cynical of all things religious, and spirituality became a non-existent aspect of life in our families.

Despite his obvious failings, I saw an old man stooped and frail, proud of who he is. A man who filed down Ford piston rings to fit an old Ronaldson Tippett water pump and designed his own swivel shelf when television first arrived. A man who cannot tolerate idleness and loves mental arithmetic. A man remembered by many as handsome, smart, and charming. He's my grandfather, largely estranged from family; I barely remember him at all. He died in July 2012, aged ninety-four. Never reuniting with his first love despite a drawer full of photos and a sparkle in his eye whenever grandma is mentioned. A sparkle not seen in June's eyes when Maurice is mentioned—sadness and bitterness long having replaced the allure of the handsome, charming man.

THE MADNESS DEEPENS

The three days Mick and I spend in alpine wilderness luxury at Cradle Mountain for his fiftieth birthday, are peaceful, death-free, and quiet, covered in snow and surrounded by wombats munching button grass. It's utterly, utterly, healing.

We take an early morning, icy walk around pristine Lake Dove, inhaling the scents of snow gums and pencil pines. The King Billy suite is a huge spacious room with a two-walled fire, giant king-size bed, walk-in shower with bench seats, and a hot tub on the deck where we brave the freezing air and falling snow to sink naked into the steaming water, watching the curious brushtail possums and beady-eyed black currawongs around us while I sip champagne. We wake in the morning to see a pademelon (a short, fat wallaby), with its little wet nose pressed against the glass door, waiting for a breakfast treat. The next fifteen minutes are spent hand-feeding carrots to Mr. Pademelon and his three friends. It's a welcome reprieve from the past few months and a chance to heal some of the rift in our relationship.

We return home without a penny to our name, getting back to the routine of work and family with a view to replenishing the empty coffers. Over the next three years, I'm in a slow decline. I haven't grieved the loss and trauma of losing my mother and sister, and I develop a chronic fear of phone calls; everyone is going to die and the phone is always the bearer of bad news.

Jamie lives with us, and I'm unravelling the god-awful financial mess he's dug himself into. The growing demands of my aging grandmother exhaust me daily. I realise I'm so worn out that my teaching days are numbered. My performance work dries up and orchestral dreams fade into oblivion. Chronic daily purging ruins my voice and I leave singing and choirs behind. The music that shaped and defined me for almost fifty years is now gone from my life.

I have no recollection—to this day—of having a care for my body. I care deeply how it looks, but not how to look after it. Blessed with good genetics, strong bones, healthy teeth, a strong immune system—I've trotted through life with barely a physical care, yet time catches us all. And purging on and off all these years has finally taken its toll. Was the sacrifice worth it? If I was thin enough, part of me says, *Shit yeah!* To be caught in eating disorder hell and lose the ability to sing, well that's just the price paid for my learned stupidity.

My children are knee-deep in the heady years of chronic teenage-hood, with all the risk-taking, rebellion, obstinacy, and fears every parent faces. Our marriage wearies and we pull apart from each other.

When my father's identical twin brother dies at the start of 2015, it's my undoing. Watching my adored father grieve yet another painful loss—his head resting momentarily on his beloved brother's coffin as he cries, "My other half is gone,"—becomes one straw too many, and I crack under the toll. I'm now officially no longer coping. I have chronic and obvious issues with depression and anxiety, my eating disorder is out of control, and I struggle with suicidal ideation day in and day out.

I never talk about the ideation until my psychologist unravels my story later in the year. That thought of wanting to be dead, when I was just nine years old, has played on and off in my head throughout my life. My failed overdose at nineteen was the only serious attempt, but many ideas have popped into my head as the years wear me down, the lure of eternal rest calling more strongly minute by minute.

Anxiety flares one day when I'm feeling trapped and start scratching my hands with my fingernails. I tear the skin off, and just like that, I become a self-harmer.

I once read nobody has any idea how much self-hatred it takes to make yourself vomit. The same is true for self-harm (although let's be honest, purging is just a type of self-harm). Happy people don't inflict pain on themselves—physical, psychological, emotional. They just don't. For many decades, I wondered why on earth anybody would, or could, run a blade across their unblemished skin, inflicting pain, misery, and permanent damage. I learn why.

Vanessa's self-harm was an absolute mystery to me. Why would such a beautiful, intelligent, creative, capable person do something so incomprehensible? I read books on the subject, try to accept, understand, and empathise, but I don't get it. I never ask her about it. I see her scars and try not to judge. In hindsight, I didn't try hard enough to understand, and I live with another regret.

My self-harm and purging escalates. Easy tools to calm or distract myself. I scratch my hands when thoughts escalate unreasonably, and deafening myself with the car stereo doesn't shut them out. When I catastrophise, I can't tell the difference between a likely, possible, maybe, unlikely, incredibly unlikely, or impossible scenario. In my head, they're all the same, so I leap to worst-case scenarios then take another flying leap. I tear the skin off my hands, and I'm focused on the here and now. I've inadvertently stumbled upon very poor mindfulness practice.

Mindfulness—the buzzword of the 21st century; I'm sure it's really fucking fabulous. But I suck at it. Stilling my thoughts is impossible. Popping them onto clouds and streams or shoving them in filing cabinets doesn't work; they just pop straight back into my head. What I find helpful is . . . [*I sat here for fifteen minutes trying to think of mental activities that help still my mental chaos; I can't think of any. I appear to have mentally failed this category*]. When I feel something real, self-harm stills my mind and stops the chaos in my head.

I graduate to pins, hiding them all over the house, car and my handbag; they're still everywhere, to be honest. Nobody takes any notice of innocent dressmaker pins in odd spots. I feel safe; if my distress levels are too high, I can calm down. If I'm unhappy or ashamed, I punish myself, controlling the flow of emotions by fishing out a pin and scratching until skin disappears and a trail of blood oozes out. It's hard work—pins aren't designed for self-harm—but I manage. I don't think of myself as a self-harmer; those people do much worse things.

Mick and I spend the month of May in Switzerland and Italy, making the most of an opportunity to stay with friends while they're still living in Geneva. I don't want to go. The trip we've planned and saved for since 2014 is now a chore to be completed, so I can get back to grandma, dad, my boys, and my students. Our time away together is a Band-Aid on our relationship wounds.

I graduate to knives. It's harder than you might think—carving into your own soft flesh with a kitchen knife. I realise all our knives need sharpening. I purchase razor blades and carve V into both wrists. V for Vanessa. I feel so close to her during the ritualistic sessions. Now I'm a true self-harmer. Now I deserve the title of shame.

People start to notice the marks and it's hard to hide or explain them away. My massage therapist is also a friend and notices the cuts. Sheree and Kirsten know and are concerned but they're aware I'm now seeing a psychologist. I quickly turn conversations around, steering them away from myself, and become adept at hiding my arms—long sleeves becoming my clothing of choice all year round. I'm becoming emo. A fifty-year-old middle-aged mother, hacking at her arms when she can't hack life. Not the most stellar moments of my life. It's truly shocking how quickly something becomes normal.

Like every other maladaptive coping behaviour I hide behind, it escalates. I cut myself at least two or three times a day—a ritualistic, self-soothing behaviour that both works and doesn't work to calm me. I nest in a quiet, calm, comfortable spot, with rugs, heaters, and my soft brown cat nearby, scented candles burning, a cup of tea, stashes of neatly folded tissues, and a good strong light. Both arms have neat cuts, in patterns of five—twenty on each arm. Always done in patterns of five. I start on my thigh occasionally—much easier to hide but not as emotionally satisfying without an easy visual reminder throughout the day. Under no circumstance do I want to suffer the ignominy of having to attend the emergency department for stitches; the shame of my husband, children, and friends knowing what I do is unbearable. I cut as long and deep as I can but rein it in enough that no medical attention is required.

Mick is lost in a flurry of worry, no idea how to care for the woman he's loved for most of his adult years. His ever-practical nature coming to the fore on occasion, but quiet observation is not his strong point. He has no idea my arms and thigh are covered in wounds. The normality of me hiding my flesh from him is the perfect subterfuge for indulging in my secret world of self-harm. Our polar opposite sleeping hours contributing to the ease of secrecy. Not everything is so easy to hide. A lifetime of non-observance doesn't improve with his age, and I rely on the fact that he won't see what he isn't told about. He's familiar with my body hatred, so keeping the lights dimmed or my hands pushed beneath my pillow or under the sheets hides any evidence. He never notices a single mark.

THAT SINKING FEELING

B eing at the centre of a nervous breakdown is a unique experience. Not one I recommend.

Energy levels plummet; no longer am I super bouncy and hyperactive. I stop sleeping. I'm completely exhausted. Disordered eating and self-harm are daily rituals. I cry and shake all the time. My heart races and I have panic attacks. My breathing is frequently ragged. I can't cope with the teensiest little stress (out of cat food? Disaster). I can't get myself to work, communicate with people, or articulate what I'm feeling. I'm sad in the same way an asthmatic is short of breath; without intervention, it's going to kill me. The future feels like a black hole of death, destruction, and disaster. The present feels like I'm drowning in mud, and the past looks like a string of bad decisions and broken dreams. I can't put on a happy face; I can't remember where I put it.

I can no longer care for myself—let alone my husband, my children, my father, my grandmother, my friends, my students, and my colleagues. A lifetime of looking out for everyone else and now I can't gather the energy to send a text message. All I can manage is to get out of bed and lie on the couch. I stop eating and hope to die.

Suicide: It's a dirty word. People are afraid of it. They don't want to hear it. Or talk about it. My first death wish, all those decades ago, has been a thought appearing on and off my entire life. Now it's an obsession. We all have a breaking point. I think people forget that. We . . . All . . . Have . . . A . . . Breaking . . . Point . . .

"I would be sad if you died."

There aren't many people it's possible to talk suicidal thoughts with. Practically nobody, really. I'm blessed, as it's quite unusual to have two such souls. My husband is an emotional rock, but something about Kirsten and Sheree allows me to trouble them with the things I can't otherwise share with my husband or understand myself. The sharing saves my life.

When the burden of being a burden becomes so burdensome the burden can no longer be borne, it's crunch time. Sheree said she would be sad if I wasn't here anymore. Those six little words, *I would be sad if you died,* keep me grounded one more day. Every day counts. When Mick travels for work, Kirsten turns up unexpectedly at my house to stay the night, fearing what might otherwise happen. I'm kept grounded another day. My life is broken into smaller and smaller moments, the future stretching so far out it has become incomprehensible. The old twelve-step adage of *one day at a time* is too overwhelming. I try to live one hour at a time, and when that is too hard, I focus minute by minute.

Gym class is the only reason I get out of bed. Sheree supervises my exercise, adjusting for physical and mental health limitations. She keeps a close eye on me and encourages me to stay after class to ask how I'm doing. It's the beginning of a beautiful friendship. The one hour a day I spend at the gym is the highlight of my day and the closest thing I feel to happiness. An hour when the chaos in my head is stilled and I can just be. The continued connection to humanity—to people who genuinely show love and concern—keeps me grounded.

My closest friends have faith in me, believe in me—and my capacity for recovery—long before I even contemplate such positivity. They care when I can't care for myself. They see me in my darkest, ugliest, most vulnerable moments—starving, depressed, self-harming, and suicidal. Sick, crying, unkempt, anxious, and panicked. The Girls, Sheree, Kerry, Emma, and my new Tassie friends. There's never an ounce of judgment crossing their faces. I am soon to learn how rare this is for those of us struggling with their mental health. They trust that my psychologist and GP are caring for my mental health and will intervene if needs be. Kirsten gets nervous and spontaneously visits if she knows Mick is away overnight. I beg them all not to tell Mick; it's my story to tell.

I feel guilty for not sharing the darkest depths of my inner world with Mick and the rest of my friends—my oldest, closest, most loving, caring, and compassionate friends. But my primary instinct is to protect them all from me, so I dish out the truth in nuggets—a little here, a little there. Slowly building a whole picture without ever divulging it all at once. I struggle to talk and come to rely on instant messaging.

Kirsten and Sheree are the cornerstones in the small circle of strength and love that holds me afloat as I crumble to pieces. From my circle of twelve, I start to experience something I've never really truly felt—acceptance.

FOOD RULE 233

Don't eat food.

THE LAMENTABLE ROCK BOTTOM

Through psychological therapies in my fifties, I learn anxiety manifests invisibly throughout my life; I simply have no words for it and tend to numb fears before they take root. I have a desperate need to be liked, a catastrophic fear of conflict, and an overwhelming fear of failure. All manifestations of unacknowledged anxiety are numbed behind excessive dieting, obsessive working, and an insatiable need to help and heal others, while running away emotionally in any capacity I can. I'm a hyperactive, confident, capable, much-loved teacher, musician, mother, wife, and friend. I'm an emotional robot.

When life's okay, I manage fears the same way I manage all my other emotions; I ignore them. Everyday life trots by, and I have no more major panic attacks, but when the sun goes down, I curl up in my pyjamas, desperate to run away from the exhaustion of human contact—no longer able to hold up the pretence of being strong and capable. My life is a lie. To calm the chaos in my head, I become adept at organising the chaos around me. I'm not adept at caring for my body.

I still have the body I was born with. It's served me faithfully all my years—despite what I've done to it. I'm blessed with strong bones, good teeth, a great immune system, and most excellent health. I am, indeed, extremely fortunate.

I wasn't however, blessed with confidence in this body. Through quirky twists of fate, I lost any perception of it as aesthetically tolerable. I can't look in the mirror with anything other than disdain and self-loathing. I no longer see my body as it actually is, my distorted perception saying size eight or twenty-eight all look the same, my voluptuous bust line enhancing any image reflected back to me.

Breasts are a quintessential mark of womanhood, and like most dictates of modern western society, many women struggle to accept their unique physical attributes. From the full double D cup struggling to be contained in my high school uniform to the mighty weight of a G cup as my half-century rolls around, I was always a buxom lass, an observation the smaller-busted women in my family commented upon with much disdain.

I vaguely recall when elastin held my ever-expanding mammaries in place. The voluminous mass spilling over bra cups with just enough firmness to display a cleavage envied by some, and wholly appreciated by my husband. Nipples pointed north and the soft pale flesh needed little encouragement to stay firmly attached to my ribcage. But like so many before me, I failed to appreciate the fast flush of youth while it still clung to me.

Time marches on, elastin disappears, the bosom goes south, and my shoulders gain a permanent indent where thick bra straps attempt the impossible on a daily basis. Breasts, once round and full, droop halfway to my belly, flattened across the top like a half-empty sack of flour. The occasional light brown freckle vastly outnumbered by streaks of white stretch marks. Shame—a constant companion to my sense of self—is most vehemently directed at these pendulous horrors.

September 2015, I deem the numbers on my scales to be vaguely acceptable and sign up for the breast reduction my mother recommended I start saving for in 1981. I wake from the surgery with a great weight lifted both literally and metaphorically from my shoulders. Breasts my husband hasn't laid eyes on for many years now on show for all and sundry. Doctors, nurses, family, and friends—anyone who wants a sneak peek at the new me. Still pale but now perky, an enviable asset for any fifty-year-old woman, now reduced to a C cup. Just a handful. Just enough. And for the first time since my breast buds burst into full bloom, I feel no shame.

Time softens the perkiness and fades the scars. Shoulder dents remain and ongoing neck pain is a reminder of the weight I carried for decades. The slumped shoulder position so common in big-boobed babes is something I'm reminded to work on by strengthening back muscles at the gym. Once upon a time, I entered clothes stores with much trepidation; women's clothing rarely accommodates large breasts. With a common cup size, clothing is easy to buy. I now have breasts that fit fashion.

Never once in all our years together has Mick ever passed judgment upon my size, shape, or appearance. He demonstrates nothing but the most loving acceptance of me at any and every weight. Scars, cellulite, and saggy, baggy boobs and butt mean nothing to him. He loves me just as I am. I know this.

He's also painfully aware of how I feel about seeing myself naked. As the scars fade, he drags me out of bed one morning to stand in front of the mirror—naked. He stands there, holding me, looking at the reflection I'm forced to gaze upon, and says, "Beautiful. Just beautiful."

I can't see what he sees—even as I surreptitiously turn my arms so the scars remain unnoticed. I see regret and disappointment—a body that betrays the passage of time and the toll that pregnancies, surgeries, and weight gain have taken. I see something completely unlikable—utterly unlovable. I can't reconcile his declaration of beauty with the sordid image reflected back at me. I don't know how. My body is a despicable vessel of shame. This rare moment of tenderness and love is not enough to keep our bond from splitting at the seams.

My inner world crumbles. My outer world is unchanged, and only those who've noticed the scars on my arms have any idea I'm falling apart. I arrive home physically and mentally exhausted each day and lose the capacity to manage our home or connect with my husband. He senses my internal turmoil and says nothing. I bury my internal turmoil and say nothing.

Unspoken resentments and two decades of taking each other for granted start tearing us apart. As we stand in the aisle of our local hardware store arguing over which new toilet seat to buy to spruce up the aging bathroom at home, Mick makes a snide comment about me in front of the salesman. It's the millionth time I've felt humiliated in public by those who claim to love me the most, but it becomes one straw too many. I burst into tears as we arrive home and say I can't do it anymore. I can't be married anymore; I want a separation. He's crying as he pulls me close, "I'm sorry. I know I'm an arsehole. I'll do whatever it takes. Anything it takes." And we stand there in the kitchen crying together.

May 2016. I've stopped eating altogether and lose 13kg in five weeks. I feel joyous with the number on the scales, but it's the only spark of happiness in my entire life. My psychologist wraps me in blankets when she sees me and suggests it might be time to consider an inpatient stay. I have severe depression, anxiety, panic attacks, and frequent daily episodes of self-harm. Suicidal ideation has turned into concrete plans that I'm fighting on an hourly basis not to implement. After my psychologist says a crisis assessment team needs to become involved if I can't guarantee my safety, I voluntarily admit myself to a private psychiatric hospital.

THE REVELATION

How low can I go?

My arms are permanently scarred. I'm constantly freezing. Constipation is so rampant I'm single-handedly keeping the laxative companies in business so I can shit once a week. I have constant reflux. Purging has ruined my singing. My eyes have permanent grey bags. My heart thumps so hard in my chest it feels like a kidnap victim trying to escape from the boot of an old car. My fingernails are brittle. Ketones make my breath stink, and I can constantly taste metal. My belly and back ache from heaving. My hair falls out in thick chunks, clogging the shower drain every day. The only redeeming grace is the decreasing amount of pain involved in leg waxing; when hair practically falls off you, it doesn't hurt much to rip it out at the roots.

It's a revelation to me that I can sink so low, lose so much, fail so miserably. This can't be real. At the stage of life when women's magazines claim I'll start accepting myself in body and soul, I reject everything I've become, lose sight of everything I've been, and cannot picture a life worth living.

I'm a teacher. I've been a natural-born teacher all my life. I can teach anybody who is willing to learn. So, if I fail to learn all the tools and tips that are generously shared with me, where does the fault lie? Why do I live in eternal battle with myself?

With so much revelation, how can I know so little?

SCALES OF JUSTICE

I am a prisoner in a cell of my own making.

Each morning, I stand upon the Scales of Justice to determine if today will be the day that I set myself free.

I can't bear the thought of not knowing my weight.

I can't bear the thought of knowing my weight.

No matter the number, I will turn the result into an excuse to indulge in disordered eating.

If I've lost weight, it won't be enough. I need to lose just a little bit more so I have leeway—when it all stacks back on.

If I've lost weight, it's because I haven't exercised enough, and my muscle has turned back to fat.

If I've lost weight, I must perpetuate the purging and restricting because that's how I lost it in the first place.

If I've lost weight, it's probably only because I'm dehydrated today or not as constipated as yesterday. It couldn't possibly be because I've actually lost a gram of fat.

If I've gained weight, it's because I'm a failure.

If I've gained weight, it's because I binged and didn't purge enough. Or restrict.

If I've gained weight, it's because I'm weak-willed and gluttonous.

If I've gained weight, I need to stop eating—just like I promised I would do yesterday and I'll promise again tomorrow.

If I've gained weight, everyone will notice how fat I am and judge every ounce of my existence.

If I've gained weight, all my clothes make me look fat—even the clothes I wore less than twenty-four hours ago.

Arbitrary boundaries and rules placed upon myself, setting me up to fail, imprisoning me in a life I didn't choose to enter but have chosen not to leave.

Each morning, I stand upon the Scales of Justice to determine if today will be the day I set myself free.

I know—deep in the deepest part of my heart and soul—the only way to set myself free is to be rid of the Scales of Justice. As long as I stand upon them in judgment of myself, I will never be free.

One day, I will be free.

CLINICAL INTERVENTION

I feel like a deer in the headlights. We're fortunate to still have the private health insurance I took out in order to have the breast reduction in 2015. Without it, admission to the private psychiatric clinic would be impossible. It offers little comfort as I arrive at reception with Mick and my suitcase and start filling in paperwork.

I farewelled the boys the previous day—a Mother's Day lunch together at home. I don't know how much they know, and I can't cope with knowing. They've sent me off with flowers and cards and accept my admission into a psychiatric hospital as just another thing that happens in life. They know I haven't eaten for weeks. It's a lonely, teary farewell with Mick as my life is handed over to the care of the hospital. He looks sad and forlorn, relieved and lost, as he's let out through the locked doors. He knows I'm safe now. Admission day is busy. I meet my psych nurse. Tour the clinic. Meet with the psychiatrist. Have an ECG. Have a physical assessment. Get blood taken. Hand over all my medications. Have my belongings searched. Set up my room. Go to lunch.

Lunch.

It's two months since I've eaten lunch, but my psychiatrist informs me if I don't start eating, I'll be involuntarily transferred to the public hospital psych ward. So, I'm faced with a choice—eat and stay or don't eat and be transferred. I pick up the fork.

There's a war in my head. *Eat. Don't eat. Stay. Don't stay. Live. Die.* I feel silent eyes boring into me, my head bowed, sitting alone at a small table by the window with my plate of hospital food. I hold the fork and stare at it. I can't make my hand move as an invisible force pushes it away. Eating will change everything. I don't want to do it. But I also have an overwhelming desire to please—to make people happy and to do as I'm told. A desire eternally at odds with my desperate need to do what I want, when I want.

Five minutes pass, and I'm still staring at the fork. Tears are streaming down my face. Surrounded by people eating food, chatting away like it's an easy thing to do. I'm alone. I feel utterly alone in a place I don't want to be, surrounded by people I don't know. My breath is ragged, caught in my throat, and I'm struggling to inhale. My face is flushed with embarrassment and shame. I don't want anyone to see me. I don't want anyone to know. A staff member asks if I'd like my nurse to sit with me. I nod silently, salty tears unceremoniously splashing onto the plate as I continue to stare at the fork.

My nurse sits down and gently encourages me. He's filled with compassion and understanding, common sense and logic. *Just take a small bite. Just one. Breathe slowly and deeply.* I feel like an idiot.

I can't stop the trembling, can't slow the breathing, but I force the fork to my mouth and swallow a tiny mouthful of food. It tastes like failure. One forkful isn't enough; I'm told to keep going. My nurse keeps the one-sided conversation going, firmly encouraging as I swallow tiny morsels of food. I'm wearing a size eight mini skirt. I'm the slimmest I've ever been in my entire life. Every calorie landing in my belly is instantly converting to fat. I love this skirt. I hate the fat. I'm terrified I'll never be able to wear the skirt again. My sense of control is evaporating with every swallow and vivid images of binges—past and future—engulf me.

I consume about a quarter of the small plate of food, the tears continuing throughout the painful ordeal. Finally, I'm allowed to stop. It's a good start, I'm informed. I take the dishes to the kitchen and head out to the common areas to be supervised for an hour. I hate every minute of it.

Knitting. Everyone in the common area seems to be knitting, chatting, and enjoying the camaraderie of a post-lunch chat. There's laughter and small talk. A few people say hello and I make minimal responses as I sink into my chair and wait out the hour. I have no words for small talk. No energy to engage in conversation. No will to share my story or learn about anyone else. I want to be silent and alone as the food I loathe settles into my belly and starts nourishing my mind and body.

I stay nearly four weeks in the clinic. Slowly settling into a routine, I begin meeting people, attending psychology sessions twice a day, and participating in all extra-curricular activities—walking to the shops, bus trips to a café, attending gym sessions when they're on and training myself when they're not. I eat three meals a day and panic every morning that today will be the day my skirt won't zip up.

Two weeks into my stay, I have a bath—a privilege that has to be earned and a luxury I adore as we have no bath at home. I soak in the huge deep tub alone with my thoughts. The hot water a soothing balm, enveloping me in a soft protective cocoon. I've been a water baby all my life, and have no recollection of learning to swim, yet there is a deep knowing that water is my friend and a comforter. Inevitably, thoughts drift to my mother and sister and all the opportunities I missed. All the mistakes I made. All the regrets and associated sadness with the loss of the close relationships I wanted, never experienced, and can now never have.

Seven years of unshed tears start spilling down my cheeks and sobs envelop me. *Where are they now? Can they hear me? Are they happy?* I can see them with Christian, angelic and perfect, stripped back to the essence of their being and not weighed down with the burdens of living. Cleansed of their mortal imperfections and flowing with the love so difficult to express in their earthly realm. I desperately miss them. I desperately miss what we never had.

I get out of the bath and try to dry myself and get dressed, but it's overwhelming; I can't do it. My knees weaken and I sink to the floor, sobbing in front of the disabled toilet, grateful for the standards of cleanliness maintained in a hospital and the rarity in which the locked bathroom with the bath is ever used. The floor is sparkling, and the toilet is pristine and sterile white. I lean against the wall, draped in a soggy towel. The evening nurse knocks on the door to see if I'm okay. I don't respond. A short time later, the key is turned and she comes in with a student nurse and we all sit on the floor in front of the toilet as I sob a sorry story of regret about my sister. I shed the tears of grief that have been brewing in my belly.

Over the next week, I sink to the floor most days, allowing tears to spill when I flop against a wall, wondering where the strength to stand has gone. I listen to the encouraging voices of compassion from my nurses as they watch me cry and reassure me that it wasn't my fault.

Mick visits almost every day. Sometimes we sit quietly, barely knowing what to say. Sometimes we're filled with all the news of the day. As the days pass by, it's easier to talk. I confess my history of self-harm, releasing another burden of shame.

Liam visits several times, keeping me company as we assemble a 1,500-piece jigsaw puzzle of Dalmatian puppies together—searching for eyes and tongues and spots that match.

"Can you pick me up and tell me how much I weigh?" I ask Liam.

"Probably. Why do you need to know?"

"Because I can't weigh myself here and I don't know if I've gained weight."

"Who cares? What does it matter?"

"I just need to know."

"Why?"

I'm relieved I've raised children who don't care about weight, but I'm still desperate to find out the magic number that determines how I feel. All my boys have taken my admission into a psychiatric institution with grace and acceptance; they just give me a hug and say get well. Conor barely visits—too busy with life and work. Jamie barely visits—never enough money to pay for petrol. Hamish comes over a few times and takes me out for a drive; my eighteen-year-old is the responsible adult supervising me. Liam visits regularly and we complete the puppy puzzle together. I can feel the compassion seeping out of his pores. I adore seeing them all. I have no idea what to say or how to explain how I got this low. I don't know how much they know, and I don't ask. They're smart young men in a savvy world; I suspect they know a lot. Jamie has seen it all before with his mother.

Winter is coming as I leave the clinic a month later—the silver birches and stone fruit trees devoid of leaves, the skies overcast, and a briskness in the air hinting at snow on Mount Wellington in the days to come. Everything is the same. Everything is different. The woman I've been all my life shattered into a million pieces and evaporated into dust. I don't know who this new, vulnerable, emotional woman is. She cries all the time. I don't know how to be me. I've been diagnosed with major depression, generalised anxiety disorder, and bulimia nervosa. I'm released into the outpatient programmes and the care of my psychologist and psychiatrist.

I wear the same skirt home.

I've spent hours with my head bent over puzzles, watching intently as puppies, houses and forests materialise piece by piece. I've met some of the most incredibly kind, compassionate, and caring people I have ever encountered. People who know what it is to feel shame, disgust, fear, and judgment—every day of their lives. Everyone's story is different and covers a large gamut of mental health issues (addiction, bipolar, post-traumatic stress, anorexia—to name a few). But there are two things we all have in common—some degree of depression and anxiety. And a depressing number of people experience judgment and ignorance regarding their diagnosis. It reminds me how incredibly fortunate I am to have a network of loving, supportive, understanding people in my adult life.

I pack my bags into the car and head home with Mick—grateful I have an understanding and accepting husband. I've read six books, eaten thirty-seven lunches, practised the flute, and made a new friend. I've become institutionalised, and there's gentle encouragement for me to get back out into the real world. Start working again. Go back to the gym. Meet my friends. Spend time with my husband and kids. Visit dad. Return to my daily trek to rural Ranelagh to assist grandma—keeping her company, doing her groceries, pegging out the washing, and demystifying telephone bills.

She's angry about my mysterious disappearance for a month and cuts me out of her will.

FOOD RULE 377

Only eat when I'm told to.

TEACHER'S END

I 'm eating as instructed by a dietitian and my psychologist. Apparently eating food improves cognitive function. So do anti-depressants. I leave the clinic and slip back into routine—working, gym-ing, wife-ing, friend-ing.

Normal life includes a daily trip to grandma's house and the emotional roller coaster of being endlessly accused of wearing the wrong clothes, tying my hair back, cutting my hair, wearing red, wearing pink, not wearing brown, wearing too much makeup, not enough, gaining weight, not having botox, eating, not eating—the familiar criticism I've endured my entire life now amplified to a deafening point. I feel like Red Riding Hood visiting the dementia wolf sneakily impersonating my grandmother.

I do everything I can to support and ease her last years as she navigates a world that has passed her by. A woman who grew up walking several miles to buy milk freshly squeezed from the cow and carrying it back in a tin pail can't wrap her head around the internet, EFTPOS, or telemarketing phone calls. She belongs to another era. She's ninety-eight years old but fiercely strong and independent, refusing to use walking aids for fear it makes her look old.

My return to her life sees all forgiven, and her daily demands upon my time rapidly increase as she becomes frail. When she assures the nurses in hospital that I'll be assisting her to go from bed to the toilet every time she needs to go, I'm forced to accept the reality of the one thing she was always adamant she didn't want—to be moved into a nursing home. My uncle and cousin are instrumental in supporting grandma's care. We find a comfortable facility that is geographically convenient for me and move her in. It feels like bring-your-granny day in primary school as we wheel her into the nursing home nestled against the Hobart rivulet with beautiful views of the Mount Wellington range to the west. Grandma doesn't understand and wonders when she'll go home. We furnish her small room with all the familiar belongings of her home—books, mirrors, sepia photographs, and geraniums. My visits with her increase, but the demands of caring decrease. She never learns of my mental health issues and never discovers the reason for my month-long disappearance.

The dementia ward of the nursing home is the saddest comedy you've ever seen. Harold strips naked and climbs into bed with unsuspecting women, assuming they're his long-dead wife. Jon can't speak English anymore and wanders around crying in Croatian all day, desperate for a hug from all and sundry. Sophia doesn't know she has dementia and is forcibly restrained from exiting with us in the lift every day. She escapes twice during grandma's eighteen months there. In the adjacent room to grandma, Maud screams in fear and desperation, holding out her bony hand with the paper-thin skin to me, wanting nothing more than some human touch and the absence of pain.

I'm offered jobs, money, land, friendship, and husbands. Petite Rose, with her air of English aristocracy, walks to the end of the corridor outside grandma's room each day, then lets off an earth-shattering fart before returning to her room. Pattie knits. Day in, day out. She's making a scarf to rival Tom Baker's iconic wardrobe item in *Doctor Who* of yesteryear. My life's busy and overwhelming. I'm doing better than before, but there's a long way to go. I visit every day, devouring packets of Arnott's biscuits to keep the lid tightly sealed on emotional overload.

Recovery is a word bandied about continuously. I'm in recovery, trying to recover, heading to recovery, relapsing, recovering. I feel like I'm on a road to somewhere and it's quite some time before I realise recovery is not a destination; it's merely a change of direction in the rabbit warren of life.

Part of my new normal includes regular psychology and psychiatry appointments, and attendance at DBT, dialectical behaviour therapy. When I'm not patiently explaining to my students how to count dotted crotchets for the umpteenth time or searching the supermarket aisles for any treat I can coerce grandma to consume, knowing it will be me who eats it, I'm memorising mnemonics that will one day teach me to regulate emotions, tolerate distress, and relate effectively in all my interpersonal relationships.

STOP DEARMAN PLEASE GIVE TIPP

I'm learning psychology talk. Quick, memorable ways to manage intense emotions and distress.

Stop | Take a step back | Observe | Proceed mindfully

Describe | Express | Assert | Reinforce | be Mindful | Appear confident | Negotiate

PhysicaL health | Eat well | Avoid substances | Sleep well | Exercise

Gentle | Interested | Validate | Easy manner

Temperature | Intense exercise | Paced breathing | Paired breathing & relaxation

While trying to gather all the psychological tricks of the trade I can possibly find, I'm also back at work. Struggling. I adore teaching. I've been at the school for thirteen years and love every single one of those girls. I can't possibly teach them any longer. I've lost my verve. Every day is *Groundhog Day*. Every minute with the girls is filled with angst and fear. What if they learn about my mental health issues? What if they see the scars? What if they discover I have an eating disorder? I'm a role model for girls during their most formative and vulnerable years; the thought of them learning who I truly am is horrifying.

Prior to my hospital admission, I knew my music days were numbered—both performing and teaching. I gave notice in April and agreed to teach until the end of the term. When my final day rolls around, I'm filled with the emotions so many of us must face—relief, sadness, regret, joy, pride, disappointment. Teaching is who I am. More than performing, practising, playing, auditioning, conducting—I am a teacher. And I've pulled the plug.

Dear Mrs Yemm, Happy birthday! I really enjoy playing flute and enjoy having a wonderful teacher that is really caring for all of her students. Thank you for the time you spend with me teaching me everything I know. I can't wait to learn more from you and start doing exams. You are very talented and should never give up on flute. I hope that you enjoy the rest of your birthday and I really appreciate that you chose to spend your birthday teaching me and all your other students.

Dear Mrs Yemm, You are so amazing, it's awesome! You have no idea how much I'm going to miss you! You're one of the nicest people I've ever met and I'm super sad you're going! I'll update you on how I'm going! I'll miss you so much!

Dear Simone. Thank you so much for being such an amazing teacher. You have quite literally taught me everything I know about flute, and you did it kindly, generously, and with a smile on your face (almost) all the time. We will all miss having you teach us, but I will look forward to seeing you around school. Thanks again!

You are amazing!!! I'll miss you sooooo much! I'll die without you!

You're the best EVER!! We're gonna miss you SO much! Make sure you enjoy life!

I leave school on my last day content with my contribution as a teacher.

I'm also employed ten hours a week doing arts administration at the school. It's a soft exit from music as I still get to see all my girls and keep up to date with everyone's worlds, without the responsibility of teaching and performing.

I have a small income, work a small number of hours, and I'm slowly redirecting all my energies into searching out a non-musical identity. After much resistance, I commence journaling in August 2016 and start a public blog focused on mental health issues in October. I finally feel the writing skills I accrued and loved during my Masters of Journalism in 2008 being utilised. When I start those first necessary and narcissistic journal entries, I have no idea they are the little seed being sown to germinate the new me.

DEAR DIARY

2016

Excerpts from my first post-clinic journaling (edited)

6 August

Still very dark thoughts running through my head . . . I decided to commit suicide before my birthday. When I first decided this, I started feeling overwhelmed with emotions and had a shocking day. However, the more I plan and organise, the more real this fantasy seems and the more control I feel I have.

9 August

That sense of happiness and contentment and peace and serenity that people talk about is such a distant obscure impossible concept that I don't imagine I would ever have it. I'm tired of feeling ashamed. Actually, I am just tired! So. Freaking. Tired.

18 August

Future . . . Still struggling with that concept. Not sure if I want to start future plans; I'm incredibly fearful they'll all fall flat. Or everyone will die and leave me. Do other people want to opt out all the time? I am so tired . . . When I picture my future, at the moment it's just an interminable journey of same same same. Running around looking after everyone until they die.

24 August

I was thinking about connections this morning—or lack thereof. I have lots of connections with lots of beautiful people but feel myself keeping a big distance. I'm socially disconnecting and socially very careful—very reticent—to divulge too much of me to any one person. And I feel alone and disconnected even though I have beautiful people I know love me. But I don't have the courage or the strength or the energy to really connect any more. I feel like I'm still in the place where I'm trying to decide whether to pull my socks up and move onwards and upwards, or accept what has been my normal comfortable, familiar place for so very, very long. Which hasn't really been very healthy, in hindsight. But it's comfortable and familiar. And I'm very tired.

8 September

I'm feeling a tad better than yesterday. I still don't have a lot of hope for the future. And I'm definitely still mind-numbingly tired! But today, just for today, I can picture myself staying alive a little while longer. I'm just playing day by day, but I think I can manage a few more at the moment.

4 October

I feel like I'm functioning fairly well in the real world. It isn't a monumental effort to chat with people or to do what needs to be done. I am enjoying the gym and even (gasp!) have ventured into the arena of housework. It has been six months since I last touched a vacuum cleaner. I am determined to make it through a little longer. But in the meantime, all I want to do is walk out my front door and keep walking forever and ever and never come back. Just walk until I drop. Somehow that feels more acceptable than anything else.

16 October

I am struggling. I don't know what's going on—could be myriad things or just absolutely nothing, or absolutely anything, really. But I know I feel sad and despondent and lethargic and listless and irrational and moody and sensitive and tetchy. And there's no real reason. And there are lots of reasons. I don't want to do anything. I feel as though my right to suicide is being taken away too much guilt and pressure and, "This too shall pass," and "It will all get better. Just wait," and now I have to just be here and do . . . what? I don't know. I dream each night of walking out the door and walking and walking and walking until I don't know what. Probably the police find a strange middle-aged woman, freezing cold, wandering along the highway, and cart her off to the emergency department for evaluation. Where I would be mortified at having caused such a fuss.

21 October

I have had a good day. I feel a sense of being lighter. Not physically lighter—because actually I'm heavier—which I'm not happy about. But spiritually lighter. More positive. No idea what is causing this turnaround, but I am definitely feeling more positive regardless. I am very uncomfortable with this positive outlook. But I guess that is something to work on. Really fearful it will be transitory, and I'll be telling everyone, *I told you so!* before I know it.

12 November

Today I feel so much better. More like me. Sometimes that's sad and irrational and overly stressed and not coping, but sometimes it's feeling energetic and engaged and having the oomph to participate in Facebook political discussions when previously I just couldn't be bothered. I still worry that a bit of stress will tip me over the edge very quickly; in fact, that's very feasible. So, either this is what real life is like for other people (really?) or I'm in a bubble of okay-ness that will burst at some time. But I have decided I don't want to live my life in fear of the burst bubble because that fear takes away my happiness in the moment. And while I confess I haven't really felt much genuine happiness for a long time, I am definitely feeling much more able to focus on positives and to see a future—which I didn't see before.

WELL THAT WAS UNEXPECTED

It's August 2016 and I've been back at work a couple of months but today totally fucking sucked. Since falling apart, arts administration has been my safe haven, and it's now shattered. Despite resigning from all teaching in April, I was to recommence teaching tomorrow until the end of the year to cover maternity leave for the new teacher. Then I got an unexpected call to jury duty which, according to the powers-that-be, could potentially interfere with my teaching. Apparently, they've been discussing me for weeks.

I received a formal email from the school informing me I won't be returning to teaching. It arrived shortly after I contacted all the parents last night to confirm lesson times—just fifteen hours before recommencing teaching. I'm embarrassed about what parents think and disappointed for my girls. I'm shocked there were conversations going on behind my back for weeks without anyone thinking to check details with me. I was left oblivious to the new arrangements as I went about my normal days, preparing to teach again. While on the one hand, it's a huge relief, on the other, I feel insulted, humiliated, ashamed, embarrassed, and distressed at the inference that I would underhandedly contact parents of my private students without permission. My heart's racing and tears are flooding. I have no desire to eat, so that's a bonus. I feel sick to the stomach.

I sit at my desk for the morning, looking bright, cheerful, and productive, remaining chatty and encouraging to the girls and taking all the blame for the mix up because I want the best for them and this isn't the new teacher's fault. Whether by design or error, I'm deeply hurt and want to resign as fast as possible. If we weren't financially going backwards, I'd be gone by now—my instinct to flee more profound than ever. There's a reason I numb emotions all the time; I can't deal with them.

I meet with my supervisor, mistakenly believing we'll be discussing differing interpretations of events. There's a misconception that I reappointed myself as flute teacher without consultation—the verbal conversations from six months prior now forgotten amidst the wash of other responsibilities. Colleagues I've worked alongside for thirteen years consider me capable of behaving deceptively and unprofessionally and it feels deeply disturbing. I manage a surprising amount of conversation before becoming emotionally overwhelmed and burst into tears. This new emotionally vulnerable Simone is ashamed and shocked at the public exposure of my inner world. I'm not familiar with exposing vulnerabilities to my closest confidantes, let alone my workplace.

"If you'd said something a week ago, I wouldn't be so upset," I manage. Trying to understand and defend my stance, knowing that a week would have meant time to explain the change to parents.

He laughs out loud, "I don't believe that for a moment."

As soggy tears stream through my makeup, I make the inevitable decision, "I don't think I can work here anymore."

"I'm sorry to hear that," he says, without an ounce of sorrow in his voice.

I disappear to the staff toilets feeling physically ill, sitting on the floor and slicing new V's into my wrists, hoping to calm down enough to resume the familiar spot at my desk and see out the day. I email HR asking for resignation protocols and how much leave I have available. At 4 p.m. the following day, I leave my desk, farewell the rest of the staff who have no idea what has gone on, and unceremoniously exit my musical career in the most undignified manner.

Despite my time in the clinic, all the psychological support and appointments before and after, and being pharmaceutically managed for depression and anxiety, I've made no progress with emotional regulation. I am so very, very tired.

At the time of my admission to the mental health unit, I had razor blades stashed all over the house, car, and my workplace—always some hidden right next to me. Some habits are hard to break.

Three weeks in the mental health unit gave me a break from the daily habit and I was taught healthier self-soothing options. I slip into a cycle of about two or three weeks self-harm free before being tipped over the edge by something and succumb to carving that V back in. Sometimes I just surrender to that overwhelming urge to punish myself. Losing my job at the school tips me back over the edge.

For everything I gain in that moment of pain or grief, shame or self-loathing, I lose a whole lot more. My body generally heals extremely well, but still, I have scars on my thigh and arms for eternity. Most will fade to silver pretty well, but close inspection will always betray my secret. I leave teaching for fear that my students will see the scars on my arms. More than three decades of teaching—gone. I leave music administration, because conflict and fear always lead to self-recrimination. There are people who know now, and I feel forever changed by that, as though they are always looking over their shoulder, checking up on me to see if I will do it again. I will never be the same person again.

WEARY & BADASS

My life starts to feel exhausting and all I want to do is sleep. I want to go to sleep and never wake up. To luxuriate in the endless bliss of nothingness. I want to be free from physical pain. Free from exhaustion. I don't want to feel worried or anxious or guilty or afraid. I don't want to be fat and old and lost and weary. I just want to rest. To slip into eternal, blissful rest.

My body is tired. I am fit and well, but I am physically exhausted. There is no reason. It just is.

My soul is tired. There is no reason. It just is.

I don't feel particularly depressed or anxious. I don't feel sad or teary or stressed or worried—no different than any other day. I just don't want to be.

My psychiatrist would say, "That's pretty fucking depressed!" because he's a straight talker and there's no confusing what he means. So, I guess I must be pretty fucking depressed. I don't feel it. I don't feel anything. I'm just terribly, terribly weary.

Recovery is progressing but suicidal ideation remains. There are days and moments when I forget why I'm supposed to be here—why I must stay and keep doing all the things for all the people all the time. I have days and weeks where, *one day at a time,* is too much; I just have to get through hour by hour. And I do. I keep putting little milestones in front of me—hanging on for an appointment, a birthday, a coffee with a friend. Tomorrow is a new day; make a new choice, then. And my mother's words echo inside my head, *never make a permanent decision during an emotional moment.*

You know what stops me the most? In those really, really dark moments—when temptation is utterly overwhelming, and every ounce of my being is focused on (the perception of) eternal bliss and endless restful oblivion? It is the people I care for that make me want to stay.

We need connections. We're social creatures. It's hearing: *Are you okay? Are you safe?* It's a friend reading more into an innocuous, *what are you doing at the moment?* text message and cancelling her clients until Mick comes home. It's looking at my children and my husband, dad and my grandmother, and knowing they've endured enough pain and loss and don't need any more. And it's those same connections that offer a glimpse of hope and light into the future. People give me purpose.

I'm still learning to deal with all the stresses that landed me in such a dark place, and I don't always get everything right. I'm in a much better place than I was but not as good a place as I could be. I struggle with purpose and hope. I struggle with disordered eating and self-harm. I haven't found my identity and haven't repaired all the damage I did to my relationships. I'm learning to prioritise my own health—occasionally—and I'm eternally grateful for the small circle of awesome people who love and care for me when I can't do it myself. I don't remember the last time I felt true joy and some days fear I'll never experience it again. I remember contentment and laughter and satisfaction and pride; I even experience them occasionally these days. But joy? I can't remember. Perhaps one day?

It took a long time to fall down the rabbit hole; I guess it will take some time to crawl back out. But I have found a way to shine a little light all by myself. I've stamped it onto my soft, white flesh.

To all intents and purposes, our family looked like a pretty normal, conservative, middle-class household when I was growing up. My parents weren't overly strict. Or lenient. They were just sort of *average.* Despite their shortcomings.

Piercing, body modifications and tattoos weren't our cup of tea. I remember dad thinking it bizarre I wanted my ears pierced at sixteen. I did it anyway. Twice.

Never in my entire life did I ever (ever, ever, ever) consider getting a tattoo. In fact, mostly I thought tattoos were ridiculous; who would do something so permanent to their body? That's certainly the message I gave my children for more than two decades. On my fifty-first birthday, I suddenly have an overwhelming urge to get a tattoo. Not as a decoration—as a statement. Not for family or friends. Not for you. A statement for me. To remind me my story isn't over yet. So, in February 2017 I get a tattoo.

I read about the semicolon project, a not-for-profit organisation raising funds and awareness for mental health. The semicolon represents an author's option not to end a sentence and has become representative of suicide prevention. I decide on a semicolon, to remind myself that despite chronic suicidal ideation—and the firm plans in place—I'm still here. As I read more, I find the phrase, *My Story Isn't Over Yet*, popping up all the time in relation to the semicolon project, and I feel a strong resonation. So, I have it tattooed on my wrist over the top of V for Vanessa. Partly for the statement and the reminder. Partly to stop me wanting to cut into my wrist. After going to the expense and effort of getting a tattoo, I don't want it ruined.

While playing around on Pinterest, I discover an eating disorder recovery symbol and want that too. So, I get the text and semicolon across my wrist with the recovery symbol on the back. All linked up with a squiggly line.

The tattoo fits nicely under my wristwatch, so if I'm out and about and meeting people who I'd rather not discuss tattoos (or mental health) with, it's easy to cover up.

Despite it being very early days (I've had a tattoo for a measly five hours as I write this. It is, in fact, still wrapped in cling wrap), I'm extremely happy. I feel like I've made a statement to myself. If days get dark, it's a visual reminder that I've been there before and made it through. I can do it again.

Mick calls me his badass inked-up babe, which is so not me. I'm not badass, and I'm not a babe. I'm usually a big baby. I did ask for numbing cream when the text was done, but to be honest, the tattoo with the numbing cream hurt more than the bits I had done today. So, tattoo pain is like real estate; it's all about location, location, location. Thankfully, I only wanted five words—not the normal 1,000+ I tend to dribble out when I close my mouth and let the fingers do the talking. Fast forward to 2019, and I now have five tattoos; apparently once you start, you can't stop. But each and every one has a powerful reminder and message for me.

Over the past few years, I've become fit, strong, and healthy. I go to the gym and treasure the support and love of all the women. I feel a sense of community and know that no matter what happens in my day or my life, I always make the time to get to gym—to connect with people and keep my body strong and functional as I travel through middle age and venture into old age. I see seventy-plus-year-old women lifting weights, rolling on fitballs, boxing, throwing medicine balls, and swinging kettlebells. They are amazing. Their lives have changed too.

Mick and I hike in the wilderness, enjoying the serenity and beauty of the natural world. I climb mountains, kayak, and hike for miles with family and friends. Nature is fantastic preventative medicine for me.

Strength and fitness become integral to my health and longevity—not for the sake of competition, getting skinny, or looking fab in Lycra, but for maintaining and improving my physical and cognitive functions and, more importantly, finding a community of women who support each other through anything. Women who strive to build each other up, not tear each other down.

THE HITS KEEP COMING

Twenty-four years. It's December 2016 and we're celebrating nearly a quarter of a century of surviving each other's shit. That's what marriage is—loving somebody enough to accept their crap and being fortunate enough to have the acceptance reciprocated.

All those times I closed down and refused to communicate. When I was so suicidal that he didn't know if I'd be there when he got home from work. All the times I spent money we didn't have, ate too much food or none at all, blamed him for my own problems, and refused to learn how to put air in my car tyres.

All those times he publicly criticised me or got angry over trivial shit. Treated me like a child. All those times he ignored what I said, dismissed my feelings, drove like a demented maniac, and left the toilet seat up.

At the start of the year, I said I couldn't do it anymore. My own mental health was so precarious, and every little marriage bump an insurmountable burden. He buried his head on my shoulder and we sobbed together again.

"I'm sorry. I'll change. I'll do whatever it takes."

I stayed. He changed. And we both did what it takes. Because for every piece of shit in our relationship, there's a huge nugget of gold. All the times he gently held me when I fell apart. When he brought me food to ensure I'd eat. When he sponged me clean in the shower after surgery. All the times he not only said he loved me but more importantly, he showed it.

We celebrate our twenty-fourth wedding anniversary with a night at a little retreat just fifteen minutes from home, hoping to heal all the rest of the hurts that have remained unsaid over the past ten months. We snuggle. We communicate openly. We have a couples massage and soak in the huge hot tub.

After dinner, I gather the courage to say we have a lot more work to do on our marriage, but I think we're going to get there. We need more open communication, and in the interests of absolute transparency, I tell him about my blog—an evolution of the private journaling I started after leaving the clinic in May and a pastime he has no idea I've been developing over the past few months. The hundreds of posts and thousands of words I've written, detailing every emotional trauma. Every fuck up. Every healing moment. All the intimate details of my eating disorder behaviours, anxiety, depression, self-harm, and suicidal ideation. Everything he's understood at a surface level, but we've never discussed. Because my capacity to speak emotional truths is sparse, but writing emotional truths is easy.

After gin, champagne, and the anticipated anniversary sex, I fall asleep in the big Victorian-era bed. Mick stays up all night reading every single post on my blog. He reads every single word. Even the posts that have nothing to do with my mental health. He reads it all, and when I wake early in the morning, he cries, reminds me how much he loves me, and thanks me for sharing myself so intimately with him—no resentment at the public sharing of my private life. We're well practiced at poor communication. The angst of the past year melts away, and we feel closer than we've ever felt before.

We get ready to go into the city for a proud parenting moment— watching Conor dressed in cap and gown graduating as an engineer and walking into adulthood with confidence and clarity. It's going to be a perfect day.

Perfection—*the perfect illusion*. A word I've been taunted with my entire life. *You're not perfect, you know.* I never thought I was.

"Oh my God! No wonder you've been so stressed!" reads the frantic text message from my cousin at 8 a.m. I have no idea what she's talking about.

While Conor revels in the joy of finishing university and moving into the next phase of his life, Liam is facing the consequences of ill-conceived decisions from a year ago—his name plastered in indelible black ink across our local newspapers; his misdemeanours made public and misrepresented, as hastily crafted news stories so often are before the justice system has its chance to weigh the pros and cons. Liam's story is not mine to tell, but on our wedding anniversary, my heart is torn apart again. I can't be in two places at once and Liam doesn't want us there. I'm with Mick and our newly repaired partnership, and we're going with Hamish to Conor's graduation; meanwhile, across the road, Liam sits alone before a magistrate. I become afraid of hope and start to crack again.

With the cracks comes the catastrophising. With the catastrophising, I start to shut down. My fatigue comes back. It went away for a while. I didn't miss it. *Good riddance,* I thought. Then it came back. *For fuck's sake,* I thought.

Now I can barely struggle out of bed to go to the bathroom. I'm still doing all the things everyone else does—get dressed, go to work, care for people, stare at the vacuum cleaner—but I don't have the energy left for anything else.

Recovery is my primary mental goal now. I must recover. I must believe it's possible. I must believe I am worthy. I will recover. I do believe it is possible. I'm working on the worthiness thing.

Fatigue is a right bastard of a thing. It really is. I know that loads of carbs won't fix it, but food is jolly comforting, and when you're too tired to watch television, eating feels like a great idea, and the problems of guilt and self-loathing you know are going to hit the moment you stop is a problem you're happy to defer. Until next time. Again. And again.

There's no easy way to fight fatigue. There's no easy way to find recovery. There's no easy way to be in recovery when you're fatigued. There's just no easy way—full stop.

FOOD RULE 610

Take teeny, tiny nibbles.

ANA'S IN TOWN

I t's 2017. A new year and I have a new job. I love it. Just a few days a week doing office management work for a performance academy. I'm bringing together my love of the arts and young people, with my obsessive organisational tendencies. It's a small company with great people and loads of gorgeous kids. For a few moments here and there, I feel happy. I even chill out enough to start reading again, finding a memoir of an eating disorder survivor.

I turn the final page and feel the familiar emotional paradox, contentment knowing the story in its entirety, and sadness leaving the world I'd inhabited. But this time a third feeling—I'm triggered. It isn't the anticipated reaction, but the page closes and I relapse. Just like that. Not into bulimia, but restriction.

It's six days since I finished the book, and my sanity has fled. I've lost nearly four kilos. I know it's idiotic. I know it's unsustainable. Yet when it comes to making choices about how, what, when, where, if to eat—it's not me in charge.

Inside the carapace plastered around my heart live two individuals. Let's give them cliché names; it's easier to remember. Ana and Mia. Mia has been prevalent virtually all my life, but Ana sneaks out to play from time to time. Ana has whipped on high heel boots and her favourite little black number and burst through that shell with a song and a dance. Legs akimbo, arms in the air, and the confident shimmer of jazz hands.

When I first restricted my food intake, I stopped eating altogether. It's not rocket science to figure out that it wouldn't last. Six weeks later, I was living in a mental health unit. Now Ana's here without her friends—*depression*, *anxiety* and *self-harm*. She feels in control. She feels euphoric.

Intellectual Simone knows rapid weight loss is muscle mass and fluids—not fat. And every period of restriction is followed by binging. I know it's not sustainable. But I'm not in charge here. Ana is. And she's partying hard.

Yesterday, I spent two hours eating a banana. Two hours. My entire life, I've eaten like a starving woman fending off rabid dogs for the last vestige of crumbs on the floor. And yesterday, I spent two hours eating a banana. It was the first food I'd eaten all day. And I felt great.

That's the restriction high. I can do what I want; you can't make me get better. You can't make me eat. And I'll prove to you that I'm in control. I'll prove to myself that I'm in control. I'm strong. I'm invincible. I am woman and I can roar.

And I can starve.

There's a little voice inside saying, "You fucking idiot. It's not gonna last, and you know it."

And Ana's staring down at me saying, "I don't care."

FOOD RULE 987

Only eat what others eat.

SELF-CARE

Self-care. Yet another modern-day buzzword.

There are over 242 words with the prefix *self* and I've nailed a few of them: self-awareness, self-control, and selflessness, as well as self-loathing, self-pity, and self-harm. But there are others I struggle with, partly because I fear becoming self-absorbed, self-serving, and selfish.

I'm repeatedly reminded that in order to become a whole person, to recover and become healthy, I must learn self-compassion, self-love, and self-care.

So, after a little self-reflection, I've worked out my personal self-care needs. From there, self-compassion may follow. I'm pretty good at hedonistic, head-in-the-sand kind of stuff, but mental health recovery needs work a lot less fun and a bit more productive. So, I make a list of steps to self-care.

Nourish my body—three times a day. With healthy food that makes me feel great—in body and in spirit. And stay hydrated. Man, that sounds so easy when I write it like that. I feel like I could write a whole book on how to eat well, but when it comes to real life, most days I can't get from breakfast to morning tea without fucking up. I've been looking at what everyone else is eating and copying them; what they eat, I eat. I need to choose my dining buddies carefully.

Exercise. I only get to the gym four days a week now, so the other three days I need to do something else. Is there a fine line between healthy exercise and overexercise? I bet there is. If I cross the line, I'm sure someone will let me know.

Mindfulness and meditation. Ten minutes a day. Twice a day sounds even better but perhaps I shouldn't make things prohibitively complicated. The practise of taking time out to check in with mind, body, and spirit—to let go of the past and future for a few moments—is no longer limited to Buddhist monks, or yogis in search of spiritual nirvana. It's mainstream practice, taught to children in schools, and discussed in workplaces, gyms, therapy, and the media. I Google benefits of meditation and mindfulness to discover 67,000 scholarly articles. I learn meditation requires taking time out to sit and focus, whereas mindfulness is paying attention at any given moment and requires no extra time in the day. It feels really important; the monkeys chattering in my head never shut up.

Rest. I'm so fucking tired. All the time. There's no mental let-up from the moment my feet hit the floor until I get back into bed at night and I need proper mental downtime. Not *Candy Crush*, Facebook, and Instagram. Not reading, writing, and worrying. But lying down, doing nothing. Apparently, other people do this kind of thing?

Stay in touch with friends. I have awesome friends. I sound like a broken record, but if there's one thing I'm grateful for, it's the people that stick by me. Yet I shy away from reaching out as it feels exhausting.

Clean my house. I can't begin to describe my hatred and horror at being in a dirty, messy house. Then I can't be bothered to clean it. I create a miserable living space and feel sad about it. This feels like a self-piteous, self-inflicted rabbit hole that I can make a proactive decision to do something about.

Spend wisely. When I'm not being self-destructive with binging, purging, restricting, or cutting, I mindlessly shop—with money we don't have. Anything at all to avoid emotions. But a delicious new pair of shoes I don't remember ordering turning up at the door weeks later causes friction between Mick and me.

Nurture my marriage. We've been together nearly twenty-five years. If nothing else, it's easier to stay and fix it than to leave and break it. We have so much history. There are so many memories. And so much love. But a quarter of a century also brings a lot of resentments, bad habits, and taking things for granted. I don't want to get divorced, so I need to work on being happy in the marriage.

Not one of these things come naturally. I'd rather punish my body, wallow in self-pity, and push myself beyond my physical capacity to do any more, than learn the basics of self-care that everyone around me seems to have at least a small handle on.

ERA'S END

June 2017. My grandmother passes away in her sleep overnight. I've been caring for her almost daily for a decade. On Tuesday, she woke, reached out to hold my hand, and said, "Thank you for everything you've done for me." They were her last words. They were kind, loving, heartfelt words. She was ninety-eight and two thirds.

She wrote this poem when I was just a few days old.

SIMONE

Where did you come from little child,
You who drive your parents wild.
What seeds long past have had their day,
In varied loves—to have their way.
A child of fire—a child of flame,
Contrary and wild but never tame.
What does the future hold for you,
Little devil tried and true.
May it bring you all things good,
Fame and fortune compassion too.
Love and pity, joy and pain,
Or your loved ones loved in vain.

Bless you little devil child,
Though you're here to drive us wild.
Without your fire we well may be,
Untried and cold—we'll wait and see.

I read this and feel the great love that was intended. I read it and wonder why the word devil is used twice to describe a beloved first grandchild. An infant—wild, contrary, and never tame. What did my grandmother see in me?

My mother had a fractious and difficult relationship with her own mother, as I went on to have a difficult and fractious relationship with these key women in my life. Like my mother, my grandmother was petite with dark curls. She was called Peace as a child. The youngest of the three formidable McDougall girls. Her sister was born in 1914 and grandma in 1918—war and peace. That wasn't her real name though. Her real name was June.

Peace suited her though. Grandma was quiet, determined, passionate, and devoted to family, the peacemaker. She leaned very strongly towards the left in her lifetime of politicking and had more than the occasional peace sign hanging around the house. Born in 1918, she eventually took to being a child of the '70s with a passion for sunflower wallpaper, cask wine, and Suzi Quatro.

When she was born, the population of Australia was just over five million, a block of land in North Sydney cost £200, and a loaf of bread just fourpence. She lived through the Great Depression, watched three monarchs crowned in Great Britain, and saw Dame Joan Sutherland live at the Hobart Town Hall. She welcomed new life into the world and farewelled most of her loved ones. Woven through the story of her life was a love of all things Scottish and indulging in an afternoon glass of watered-down cask wine. She was born into an era where electricity, running water, and motor vehicles were rarities. Those new-fangled things came later in her life, but as a young girl, she used candlelight and kerosene lamps, carted buckets from the well, and spent most of her early years with horses and carts. If they ran out of milk, she walked a few miles to the neighbours with a bucket in hand, squeezed a little out of old Daisy, then walked home again. They were simple times, and they were active. As a result, she was a petite, fit, healthy woman. Being overweight was not something she could comprehend—or accept. Being fat was something she always felt compelled to comment upon.

Now it's 2017, and I've lost grandma. It's both a blessing and a curse. Her demands have been huge and worn me down. Emotionally, she's torn me to shreds. But every piece of the framework that keeps me anchored to this earth is slowly being torn away. Another solid strut, gone.

I was so close to my grandmother as a child. My brother and sister were only a year apart and a hyperactive handful, so I often stayed with her for weeks at a time. She spent her entire life taking in not just grandchildren but orphaned animals, stray and orphaned women and children, and almost anyone in need of a place to stay. Her door was always open, a spare bed always found, no matter the day or time. Despite a lifetime of financial scarcity, her table was never empty, and all were welcome to share what she had. She was a champion of lost children and women.

In her ninety-eight years, she led a simple life—reluctantly travelling interstate to visit family and never going overseas. She worked as a milliner before marriage and children, then devoted her life to raising her own children and any others that crossed her path. She could nurture any plant and turned bare dirt into a veritable rainforest while caring for a menagerie of cats, dogs, birds, fish, horses, wombats, and all creatures great and small. She gave up smoking more times than anyone I know—finally giving up permanently in her eighties—and ate simply. She was blessed with excellent health and longevity, a sharp mind and quick wit. From my grandmother, I inherited a great love of reading and an appreciation for writing. I know if she were here today, while she would never say it out loud, she'd be incredibly proud of me for penning this memoir.

Grandma wasn't blessed with an innate and empathetic understanding of others' emotions and feelings. Many of the dysfunctional lessons my mother inadvertently taught me as a child were passed down by her own mother. Completing the familial feminine trilogy of chronic criticism was my baby sister Vanessa—the third petite, dark-haired woman I was unable to measure up against. While heavy emphasis was always placed on the importance of looks and appearance, it was made abundantly clear that I couldn't measure up. I learned that I wasn't good enough. Whatever that actually means. No matter how old we get, or how much compassion and love we develop for those who inadvertently destroyed our self-worth, it's a lifetime's work to learn to say, *I'm good enough*. Yet despite their failings, my familial trilogy is gone, and I desperately mourn the loss. I've watched the breath pass from my mother, my sister, and my grandmother. *It's not fair,* I want to scream to the rafters.

Where are they now? Are they cleansed of all their flaws and shining like angels? Watching over me? That's what I choose to believe. They are together. Reunited. Three women—incapable of expressing true love. Desperate for love and connection. Now reconnected. Grandma, I love you, and I miss you. Thank you for all the dead plants you resurrected and the nearly dead chickens you nursed back to good health. Thank you for a lifetime's memories of puppies, kittens, gardens, and sunshine. Thank you for the babysitting and the company and for always being there. Thank you for the books and the love of nature. May you be at peace. May you be with your cherished family.

FOOD RULE 1,597

Only eat at night.

THE TUMULTUOUS RIDE

It's December 2017, and this time we're celebrating twenty-five years of marriage. I go all out, spend money we don't have, and book us onto a cruise in the South Pacific. Knowing Mick's intolerance for crowds and my anxiety with strangers, I book a junior suite. Just weeks before departure, the cruise company upgrades us to a penthouse suite, replete with chocolates and champagne, an enormous balcony, two marble bathrooms, freshly laundered clothes upon request, and afternoon teas in our living area. We're spoiled rotten for ten days, experiencing a juxtaposition of VIP life, and guilt at having nice young men come in and tidy our shoes in the walk-in wardrobe every day.

After twenty-five years of marriage, it's hard to come up with interesting gift ideas; a lot of time we don't even bother any more. Under the influence of a bottle of free champagne on the ship, I decide on something I perhaps wouldn't consider when entirely sober. I make an appointment for a Brazilian wax. *You'll never look back!* the girls' say. Yeah, right.

I rock up the next day—completely sober—wondering what the fuck I've signed myself up for. Let's just remember for a moment that I am a lass with fairly significant body image issues, so baring my lily-white ass to a complete stranger is an anxiety-inducing event of epic proportions. Nonetheless, I want to surprise Mick, so I step out of my shorts and knickers while a lovely young woman asks how thick my forest is. *Umm . . . Not too bad?* I have no idea really—having nothing to compare it to.

I lie on my back, naked from the waist down. The nice young girl gets wax strips, pressing them into my apparently sparse forest before ripping them out in one swift motion.

We chat about all sorts of stuff that has nothing to do with pain and indignity so both of us can pretend we're catching up over a nice latte. Then I bend one knee right out to the side—so she can get a good close look at my lady parts. Now that we're getting to sensitive areas, she applies hot melted wax rather than strips. She periodically tests the wax to see if it's cooled, then rips those bits out too. Once the forest is denuded on that side, it's the other knee out. All good so far. I lift my legs into the air, hug my knees, and pull them back as tight as I can. I make a mental note not to ask if she can see my haemorrhoids and I'm grateful for my hypermobility. She rips out the last of the hairy patches, then finishes the job by finding a pair of tweezers to pluck out errant pubes that refused to be evicted with the rest of their friends.

Twenty minutes after we begin, I'm having talcum powder gently patted onto my now completely bare privates. I have no recollection of the last time talcum powder was applied down there, but let's just assume it's been over fifty years. Later that evening, Mick discovers how I spent my afternoon. It was a surprise anniversary gift indeed.

Something that is not a surprise is my continued difficulty with food. It's over a month since our anniversary cruise came to an end and the real world just settles right back in. I have an unerring swing from starvation to binging and the endless purging that goes on regardless of the pendulum. I'm currently only eating when Mick watches me, and that's almost exclusively at night. My self-care plan from last month has flown out the window—along with so many other plans. My beautiful psychologist suggests I consider a specialised eating disorder inpatient treatment programme.

We talk about the tumultuous highs and lows of the past month; there were some lovely positives and some not so lovely sunken depths, and for the first time, she suggests a specialist clinic.

I'm afraid everything will be fantastic while I'm incarcerated then when I'm back in the real world the bubble will burst and it's back to square one.

I'm afraid I'll be the only old person in a sea of teenagers.

I'm afraid I'll be the only fat person in a sea of anorexics.

I'm also cognisant of some positives.

I can surrender all responsibility for my eating to trusted professionals.

I'm told my weight should stabilise (as should my bowel function and all the other parts of my body not enjoying this wild ride).

My friends and family will get a rest from my insanity.

I feel hopeful just at the thought of being an inpatient. At least if I fail as an inpatient, I'll know I've tried everything. I research clinics and narrow it down to four options—all interstate, as there are none in Tasmania. I don't know anyone in real life who's been down this path, but I'm open to the concept. It feels like a chance.

I need a referral and a vacant bed. They're like job security—pretty jolly hard to find. I fly interstate to visit an admitting psychiatrist at my preferred clinic. So off I dutifully trot—full of hope. Foolish me. Hope is quickly quelled—as hope so often is. I'm not sure why I'm hellbent on going into hospital, but as soon as he suggests I trial a drug for a month before considering inpatient, I get teary and sulk. I pay the bill, then promptly catch an Uber to the airport, order McDonald's—food I eschew under normal circumstances—then scoff it at lightning speed before throwing it all up. I buy four Krispy Kremes and eat them sitting on the toilet in the ladies room. I throw those up too.

I'm knee-deep in punishment mode. I go home with a prescription for a new drug that apparently works on compulsive behaviours and has the added bonus of reducing migraines and aiding sleep. Two side effects for which I'll be very grateful. I have no faith whatsoever that a pill can miraculously change me.

I try to process my negative response to the doctor's suggestion and shamefully realise a lot of it's to do with not getting my own way. It pains me to say it, but it's true. I'm a fifty-one-year-old toddler. I put a lot of expectations, hopes, and plans into the hospital stay, and for them to be postponed or cancelled is not easy to take. I want to live without an eating disorder. You have no idea how badly I want that. I dreamt going into hospital was the answer, and to be told a pill is a better option is a very bitter pill to swallow. I've taken two so far and there have been no miracles. I am, in fact, in a cycle of horrendous binging and purging—as though I need to prove the psychiatrist wrong.

Compulsions are a major problem for me, and this drug has been chosen as one that can apparently target compulsions. I can't conceive how that works, but I don't need to understand it. I just need to swallow the pills.

If I could abdicate responsibility for food decisions for the rest of my life, I would do so right now. Right this minute. There's so much angst involved in food. I desperately desire food and simultaneously hate every morsel of it.

It takes less than a week before the miracle drug knocks me around. This morning, I couldn't for the life of me work out what year it was. I don't mean 2017 or 2018. I didn't know if it was 2000, 2008, 2020. I had no idea and was utterly confused. When I asked Mick what year it is, he looked at me with a very familiar, *you have two heads*, kind of look. "Well, it's not 2017 anymore," and then it all clicks back into place, and I know when we are. But for a moment, it was panic stations. I hate this drug. In under two weeks, I become one of the few bulimics my very experienced psychiatrist has had that reacts extremely badly, and I'm given an inpatient admission date in two weeks' time.

I want to starve myself until I get there—to be as thin as possible before they make me eat food all the time. I was hoping to throw up my two bowls of cereal this morning, but I wasn't quick enough, and they went down too easily. I strategically swallowed a spoonful of peanut butter before lunch because it will block the lap band and I'll throw everything up. Which I did. A lot. Ditto for dinner—a bigger binge followed by forty-five minutes of trying to get rid of it all. The inside of my throat feels like razor blades. Can't eat for fear of getting fat. Can't stop eating because I'm a pig. All the gazillions of times I've tried the moderation thing, or the make lists of rules thing, or follow what other people say thing, or just let myself eat when I feel like it thing, or follow my body's signals thing—none of it ever makes a scrap of difference. I binge or starve. Every time. And I hate myself every time I eat food. I've been binging my entire life. I don't recall not binging. The purging has been intermittent and restarted after the lap band—surgical bulimia. I keep telling myself I would sooner be dead than fat.

But I don't ever want to purge again; it really sucks. It tears my throat out and the heaving hurts my belly. And I don't want to damage the lap band. Rather than starve or binge tomorrow, I want to be a minimalist. Cup of tea for breakfast. Something tiny at lunch. Then eat food with friends or my husband tomorrow when they're watching to see if I eat.

Now, I have just two days left to endure before all control over food is taken away from me and that's the bit I'm looking forward to. Six weeks without angst over if/when/how/what/why I should eat. Six whole weeks where I'm not in charge.

THE EXODUS

Dear Simone,

Thank you for taking the opportunity to read this letter. I appreciate that it is going to be confronting but unfortunately there are times when we need to hear a difficult truth; without acceptance of the facts, we cannot make changes and move forward.

Simone, I was here before your exodus from the comfort of your mother's womb. I have protected you from the elements, given shelter to your organs so you may grow and function in the way you were designed to be. And I have wrapped you in a layer of protection from illness and harm. I am here for you and always have been.

In return, you have intermittently starved me—forcing metabolic changes that benefited neither of us and psychological distress that has brought you to your knees. You have alternately binged and purged the very nutrients designed to nourish and protect, then berated me for perceived failures.

You've cursed your damaged vocal cords, developed brittle hair and nails, and succumbed to chronic malnutrition and eternal constipation, all while knowing deep in your heart that you're damaging the very body you so desperately want to control.

You've looked in the mirror and scorned every inch of my being. You've undertaken surgeries that have scarred your body and soul in an effort to fix an internal problem with an external solution. I am now scarred from head to toe. But Simone, have courage. I am resilient. If you learn to trust me, I can deliver on the health you not only desire but deserve. Let's begin anew—working with each other rather than against.

Kind regards,
Your Body

COMING OF THE DAWN

January 2018

Extracts from my private journal entries

My world has become very small.

I have a bedroom. There's a communal area where we eat and watch television. There's a corridor and people.

I can see the rest of you outside the window—wandering around with your freedom and day-to-day worries. Not limited by regimented clothing guidelines and eating structures. I see you. I envy you. It's not your ability to walk out in the fresh air I envy; I can discharge from here any time I choose. What I envy is your normality. Your decision to eat what you want, when you want. I envy those who don't stress and ruminate about those choices every moment of the day. I long to be just like you.

Day One: What have I done? I'm a fish out of water. I'm so far out of my comfort zone, I can't see where it is any more. This is the single most foreign environment I've ever been in. I hope it's worth it. The fact I feel so uncomfortable is surely a good thing. If it was easy, comfortable, and familiar, there'd be nothing to learn. Mick and I have never been apart for six weeks, and I wonder how it will affect us. I wish I wasn't in this boat, but now that I'm in it, I hope this is a safe harbour. It has to make a difference; it's a huge upheaval for my family. And I'm tired. I'm so tired of this shit, and I don't want to do it anymore. The psychiatrist inferred my goal of normal eating is not absurd or unrealistic. I repeated my history endlessly today—dietitian, nursing manager, care nurses, psychiatrists— and I'm shocked by how shocked they seem. Is my story so unusual? I've survived four meals—kept them all down. Feel completely bamboozled by lots of stuff. It's going to be an interesting stint. Onwards and upwards. One day down—forty-one to go.

Day Two: No better than yesterday. I'm still a landlocked fish. Compared to the clinic in 2016, it's impersonal and unfriendly. The girls are lovely, but there's little socialising. Meals are a silent, sombre affair. A lot of the programme is about normalising eating, but apparently only in the sense of regular, nutritional intake. There's absolutely nothing normal or enjoyable about the way we eat. At handover, the day nurse told my new nurse, "Simone has been really anxious today," which wasn't something she'd mentioned to me. I'm surprised she noticed. When I lined up for meds this evening, she commented on how incredibly anxious I seemed at dinner. I did? I kept all food down. Lunch was problematic and took two hours to get through the lap band, but I managed. I could easily have thrown it up after the supervision and briefly considered it, but I'm not here to play games, so if I can keep it down, I will keep it down. Which generates a lot of mixed feelings—*gonna get fat, not gonna purge any more, but I'm getting fat, not gonna purge any more, I hate food, not gonna purge, this too shall pass, not here to play games.*

Day Three: Massive fail. I meticulously kept all food down, despite discomfort and difficulty. After talking to the dietitian, I decided to have ice cream for supper. I dished it up, then stared at it, and couldn't do it. Felt so ashamed—all these young girls around and I'm staring at a bowl of ice cream like it's going to kill me. And the thoughts racing through my head—*I can't eat this, I'll get fat, I'll binge, it's bad food, I can't eat this, I'm not a normal person, I've eaten ice cream thousands of times, this is no different, just suck it up princess, why am I here, I want to go home, I can't eat ice cream, I don't deserve it.* All the while, I'm scratching at my hands to stay grounded and hoping the floor would swallow me up and I'd drop dead. I couldn't eat the ice cream and was given a supplement instead. It's like a chocolate milkshake somebody ruined. I didn't want that either. So humiliating—a middle-aged woman panicking at the sight of ice cream. Nobody says anything. Nobody will say anything. Just my lovely nurse who sat with me the whole time. I feel so old. There's nobody here with my longevity of eating issues, and I don't know recovered people with my kind of history. It leaves me without hope or faith that change is achievable even though people keep telling me it is. Without hope, I can't do this process.

Day Four: What a mess. I'm at war with myself. The metaphorical *they* say things get worse before they get better. Now I have to see how much worse and for how much longer. I threw up at afternoon tea time. I was desperately trying not to, but the lap band pain from the blocked food was overwhelming, and I was going to spontaneously vomit if I didn't purge. Nurses kept saying, "Stay calm. Deep breaths," but what the fuck will that do? I had food blocked up from belly to breast and it couldn't go down. They think I'm playing games—that I'm using the band as an excuse. I'm not. Or if I am, I'm completely unaware of it. It's not intentional. All the other things can go wrong, but I want a clean slate of no purging, and now it's ruined. It makes me want to give up. Why did I throw up? Because I unexpectedly found six Brussels sprouts on my lunchtime plate. The moment I saw them, I knew they wouldn't stay down, but I didn't know what to do. Three hours later, I had a glass of water and a mouthful of custard, then thought I'd vomit at the table, so I left and lay down on the floor where I promptly tried to sink so deep into the beanbags nobody would ever find me again. I'm mortified having so much attention on me. I wanted to go to my room and be miserable on my own. It wasn't allowed. I wanted to walk around to see if the food could go down. Not allowed. I moaned and groaned and rolled around in distress until I couldn't keep it in then raced to the toilet. With an overwhelming sense of relief—coupled with disgust and disappointment. After that, I was given meds because they're concerned about my anxiety levels. Which I'll concede are sky-high. But having Brussels sprouts stuck in your lap band is not conducive to relieving anxiety. I've spent most of today and yesterday crying. It seems like the day three post-birth hormonal surge when your milk comes in—inevitable. I don't know how to deal with everything. The processes and procedures are foreign, and I don't know what to expect. Nobody says anything. I trot along to meals and groups and that's it. Nurses do handover and seem to know all about me even if I haven't spent a single moment with them. I don't know how to face tomorrow; I just feel like an abject failure. But tomorrow will come regardless of my desires and face it I will have to. I've said *no Brussels sprouts on all future menu plans*, so that's one less problem.

Day Five: Despite being repeatedly told I'm not an abject failure, I feel I am. Perhaps perspective will hit down the track, but right now things aren't progressing as expected or in any sustainable way. I threw lunch up again. I thought it would be okay. It wasn't. I rolled around in misery in my bedroom, hugging a pillow, with a vomit bag in hand just in case. In the end, I gave up and went to the toilet to purge. Have chatted extensively today with the nurse and the dietitian. They're kind and understanding— which is more comforting than yesterday. Nonetheless, I'm struggling with mood and anxiety. I'm constantly tempted to tear my hands to pieces and have managed to produce a few obvious grazes from scratching. Found a paper clip and started to carve away but thought better of it. Lovely nurse has asked me to find her (or anyone) any time I need to hurt myself. Easy to say. Logic doesn't come to the fore when I'm distressed, and with the eating disorder kicking, fighting, and being subjugated, self-harm wants to come back and play to fill in the void. There are two little angels sitting on my shoulder. They're perfect, beautiful, golden, and cherubic, with wings of gossamer. One is the devil in disguise, and I can't tell which. They look the same and speak with a voice full of wisdom and compassion. I told this to the dietitian, and she said that's why I'm here—for other people to tell me what to do and to shut that disguised angel up. I stared at dinner in tears, tearing up my fingers because I'm terrified food will get stuck. So, I had yet another supplement. I have no idea what the other girls think, and I'm repeatedly told it's none of their business what I do, and none of my business what they think. Not a lesson I've learned but one I appreciate.

Day Six: I'm completely and utterly drained. Woke early for my weigh-in (no details even though I'm itching to know). Had a lovely time writing a letter to my vagina in our morning therapy group. Breakfast, morning tea, lunch, and afternoon tea were all a breeze. I was careful, and there were no complications. My cousin visited, so I felt special and less isolated, more loved and cared for. Then the news came through that they're renovating my end of the ward, so I moved rooms to one that is bigger, brighter, and has its own bathroom. I'm in heaven! I was given strict instructions that if I purge, I lose the room. Noted. I have zero desire to purge anyway. Went to dinner. Fish, rice, broccoli, beans, and mashed potato. It looked fine. I ate it painstakingly slowly. Two hours later, supper time is approaching, and dinner hasn't gone down. I drink chamomile tea to get things flowing. Then a glass of water and all hell broke loose. I was horridly stuck. Pain, nausea, pressure in my chest and back. I paced in my room for twenty minutes—desperate to get the food down. I found the NUM and told her dinner was completely stuck and water wouldn't stay down. She said if I didn't turn up to supper, I'd have to have a supplement at 8:15 p.m. I did point out that if I couldn't keep water down, I wouldn't keep a supplement down. Turn up or I was breaking all the rules. I went back to my room clutching a sick bag and my stomach, floods of tears, pacing like there was no tomorrow. After a few minutes, the pain was intense, and I spontaneously vomited back the water and tea. No food—it was wedged in tight. At 8:15 p.m. I was escorted to the dining room for the supplement and told to relax and drink slowly. I was sobbing and petrified of throwing up in the dining room. Another nurse sat with me and could see that with every sip, I was closer to vomiting, so she took it away. I kept saying, "It's blocked. I can't keep water down. I don't know what to do." She led me to the beanbags and got my fluffy blanket and told me to relax. I was sobbing, in a ton of pain, and desperately trying not to throw up. After thirty minutes of post-supper supervision, the NUM asked if I wanted to go back to my room. Yes, of course I do. She helped me up because by then I was horribly wobbly on my feet. She asked if I wanted my meds. No point—can't keep them down. She asked what I'd do at home when blocked. Purge. She said I'd done a great job—giving the supplement a try and not purging. I wanted to walk around—not allowed. She said she would pass a message to the psychiatrist about how hard I'm trying not to purge. I curled up in bed for half an hour, willing the food down and desperately hoping it would resolve. I walked a little and felt okay, so tested some water. Went down fine. Downed four more glasses. At one point, I could feel whatever was blocked move a little. I'm so paranoid they'll kick me out for being difficult and not following the programme. I desperately want to do everything they say, but when the band is blocked, I don't know what to do. There's going to be increasing pressure for me to get the band loosened—or worse still, emptied. I'm paranoid about having that done, as the moment I get home I fear losing all control. But I also acknowledge that's three days of genuinely trying very hard to eat well for the band, and it stuck anyway. I don't know what to do. And I'm so fricking tired.

Day Seven: Zonked. Don't know what to write. Have kept all meals down and fairly comfortably at that. They've increased my anxiety meds. Keeps me super calm, relaxed, sleepy, foggy, and wobbly on my feet. Might have helped with the food staying down that I was paranoid and ate at a snail's pace. Whatever the cause, it's been successful, and I've kept all six meals down today. I do my three therapy sessions per day, and despite my hatred of art therapy, I get a lot out of it. My depression has bloomed and is overwhelming me. I spent half of today mapping out end-it-all scenarios. Too hard to overdose—although if allowed on leave, I can buy whatever I want and do as I please. Which makes me think I need to feel a little more stable before heading off on my own. I've got Band-aids for tonight, to stop me picking at self-inflicted scratches and stop them weeping all over my bedsheets. Today my mood is pitifully low. I feel like a wild horse that's been corralled. The eating disorder is bucking, kicking, and screaming, and there's a little spark of common sense that knows this is all part of the process, and if I keep trusting and accepting it, I'll be tamed and calmed. The picture is impossible to visualise right now. I stared out my window and wondered how to get to the roof of the building over the road. I'm sure I wouldn't, but it was a lovely dream. Just to think of ending. Not going through any more hell. I think, for the most part, I'm safe—just a very down and teary day. They've managed to wrap a harness around this wild horse, and it feels foreign and uncomfortable, and I don't know how to handle it. But I've heard time heals all wounds, so it's time I need. I've slept most of today. I hope I wake tomorrow feeling less down, because I'm tired of this. I just want to get better, and I don't feel it's happening yet. I've been here a week and got worse. Is that normal? I'm very grateful I love so many of the staff, and if I choose to reach out, there's always someone there. Unfortunately, I never know what to say.

Day Ten: It pains me to say this, but I'm in a rapid downhill spiral. Perhaps this is a normal part of the process. Perhaps it's failing to meet unrealistic expectations in a relatively short period of time. Perhaps it simply just is. My depression has escalated rapidly, and I feel highly suicidal. I've been making perfectly logical plans. I mentioned this to the registrars who agreed I stay in phase one, meaning I can go out twice a week but need to be escorted. There's a certain amount of relief in this as I can abdicate responsibility for myself. I feel so far away from friends and family; it's easy to lose a sense of connection. Today, they moved me to yet another room which plunged me into a really sorrowful pity party. It's tiny and dark, has no view, and no bathroom. I feel like I'm being punished, but I don't know why. Talk to people, I'm told. I have no words. The pain is speechless and inexplicable. I couldn't eat dinner tonight—just stared at it with tears streaming down my face, then had the supplement. This endless circle of failure. I think the meds are helping; I'm more relaxed at meals although equally teary. But food is staying down more easily. I'm a complete zombie. I'd like to stay in bed and never leave. At the end of the day, I'm in the right place; I know this. But I'm miserable as all hell and I've made no progress.

Day Eleven: Exhausted. Depressed. Alone and disconnected. Hopeless. Fearful. Pointless. These are the thoughts that have preoccupied me for days. I awake in tears, afraid to face another day. Afraid I'm going to fail at this recovery business, letting down all the people who are cheering for me back home. But today I feel a small shift. Just a few little things that remind me I'm not alone. I have a powerful image of a scene from *Harry Potter* where he's about to confront Lord Voldemort, but suddenly all the spirits of his loved ones surround him. They form a protective circle around Harry and Voldemort and while Harry has to wield the wand alone, the support and love from his friends and family tip the balance in his favour, and ultimately Voldemort is vanquished. Despite feeling so far from home, I can sense Mick and my boys, dad and my close friends, all holding a safe space for me. The image is very powerful and comforting when I feel so incredibly isolated and lost. Sheree Facetimed me today, and that was gorgeous. I felt so much more connected to real life. I talked Mick through how to Facetime, and we chatted for half an hour after dinner. It was awesome. The more connection I feel, the less obsessed I am with trekking to the pharmacy to purchase an overdose. It's so easy to become institutionalised. I have to remind myself this is a small blip. While I can't say I feel great at the moment, I can definitely say it's an improvement compared to yesterday. So, I'm going to count that as progress.

Day Thirteen: Backwards, forwards, or just plain stagnant? I can't tell. I've been beaten down by the lap band and ready to have it loosened. It can't happen right now. I have to wait for doctors to talk to nurses to talk to doctors so decisions can be made. In the meantime, I stare at these enormous meals with full knowledge that they won't stay down, and after hours of pain and discomfort, when it finally comes back up, I'm told it's my mindset and I need to relax—to let the food digest slowly and take my time and it will all be fine. Not one of these people has a lap band. Sometimes when it's completely blocked, I'm asked if I'd like a tablet for the nausea. Of course, I can't take a fucking tablet; my lap band is blocked. I spent an hour today with a sick bag bringing up bits and pieces. I feel so misunderstood and out of my depth. I cannot keep down the types of food available at lunch and dinner. I cannot get the volumes in. I don't know what to do. This band will be loosened, but not today and not tomorrow, and each day there are more black marks against my name for being non-compliant when all I desperately want to do is comply with the programme. I'm here to learn, be guided and changed, and go through whatever misery needs to be gone through, but I struggle with the absolute inflexibility of the lap band. I'm terrified I'll be kicked out of the programme. There's been a contract drawn up discussing self-harm and purging. One incident of self-harm or purging will see me immediately discharged. The sense of failure would be overwhelming. The loss of hope. I need to be here and learn the skills required to conquer disordered thinking. I can't bear the shame of rejection or the sense of failure. I'm so very, very tired of crying. I want a day where there's a sense of success and achievement—something I can take home and maintain long term. I want a life, and there are moments where I feel it slipping away. I went out this afternoon and got a new tattoo—angel wings and the text, *stalked by demons. guarded by angels.* There's too much stalking and not enough guarding right now. The angel wings look like sperm. Maybe one day I can make them more angelic. I don't recall having this level of depression and anxiety for quite some time. I bought myself an anxiety bunny, something to keep my hands busy when I need to scratch. It says jellycat on the tag, but Sheree felt Hope is a better name, so I'm going with Hope.

Day Fifteen: I've been here two full weeks. I've missed eight gym classes. Two family dinners. Two Saturday morning liaisons with Mick. I've missed a thousand snuggles with my cat and countless coffees and walks with friends. I've missed work and egg sandwiches with my dad. I've missed all the worries and stresses my friends are experiencing. I've missed every aspect of my life. For what? I've cried a gazillion tears and given up trying to make the nurses understand how the lap band is restricting me because it's *all in my head.* I'm more depressed than I've been for so long. Desperate, desolate, and misunderstood. I feel so alone. I've reached out and started talking to the girls here. I'm afraid to get too close as I have no strength for anyone else's burdens. Anxiety isn't great but I've stopped scratching. My bunny is very helpful, keeping my hands busy. If I look like a fifty-one-year-old toddler, I don't really care. Hope is calming and grounding, and right now, that's a good thing. I want to reduce these mind-numbing drugs as they make it too hard to work and write. But when I don't take them, my anxiety becomes unbearable. So, it's that old rock and a hard place conundrum. I'm toying with the idea of emailing my boss and resigning from work completely, as I could be here for months not weeks.

Day Seventeen: Wow. What a day. Some corner turning happening here. If I'm not careful, I might get dizzy. Firstly, and most importantly, my baby turns nineteen today. He's not a baby anymore; he considers himself a young man, but he'll always be my baby. He sent me a photo of himself with his new coffee machine, saying "Thank you, Mumma." I'm sad I'm not there to celebrate, but super proud of the young man he's growing up to be. Almost as exciting as my baby's birthday was my visit to the bariatric surgeon. My lap band has now been drained of all fluid. I'm a free woman. Even an empty band offers a certain amount of restriction and deeply reduces hunger signals, but I should be in a much better position to eat all the foods I'm presented with. Dinner went down quite easily; I still felt enormously full with a serving size deemed to be small (doesn't look small to me). But as long as I don't rush, there's no sensation of feeling stuck. I can't even begin to express how much of a relief that is. Now that the brick wall of the lap band is out of the way, I can focus more on the origins of the eating disorder. The team here believe it's completely possible for me to find full recovery; I simply need to commit to the programme—the good, the bad, and the ugly. I'm not here to feel comfortable, make friends, or stick to things I'm good at. I'm doing art therapy (*blergh*) where I'm exploring hidden emotions and connections without even realising it. I attend DBT sessions where all the old tools are presented in new ways. I've started to connect with the other girls and share a little of our lives without sharing too much of our stories, as that isn't permissible. The biggest thing today though? I haven't cried. That's the first time in seventeen days. I continue to feel in my heart of hearts that no matter how tough it is here, I'm finally in the right place at the right time. And I owe a mountain of thanks to all those people who supported and encouraged me to make this seemingly impossible decision.

Day Twenty-Two: Today, I'm afraid of recovery. I've been in this place before—where I've felt the beginnings of change, then become overwhelmed with the fear of that change and what it might herald. So, I rush back to the safe and familiar. I ate all my meals but mentally struggled a little more with each one—as if I'm not deserving of recovery. Girls who've been here longer than me struggle so much more. At dinner, I stared at my plate of food and didn't want it. I feel so fat even though I'm assured my weight is stable, but most of the other patients are tiny. I got through the meal—slightly overtime, but finished nonetheless. Despite the band being empty, there's sufficient restriction that food goes down slowly and could potentially get stuck. After two hours, I suddenly had an overwhelming urge to purge. I could easily have done it; nobody would know. Except me. It's the strongest urge I've had since I came in. I could also easily get the food to go down if I sat up, paced a little, and had a hot cup of tea. I briefly considered my options, then boiled the kettle and found my favourite nurse. I finished my cup of tea, we had a chat, and the urge diminished. I could still purge now, but more food has passed through the band; I can feel it gurgling down. In twenty minutes, it will be supper time, and my safest option will be a drink—which is permissible. I'll have to face that choice shortly. But tonight, the eating disorder voice is yelling loudly and wanting to rid my body of this food. I can't bear the thought of getting fat again. Nor can I bear the thought of going backwards and letting down all my friends and family who so desperately want me to overcome diseased thinking permeating every aspect of my life. Today, I'm bone tired, which is hard to acknowledge when all I do is eat, rest, and write in journals. It's not exactly physically taxing. I desperately miss exercising and would love nothing better than to put on my gym gear and run down to the park right now. Not allowed. I have to allow my body to find its natural equilibrium without exercise. I'm more sedentary than a dying lady in a nursing home. I'll need to check my butt for bedsores soon.

Day Twenty-Five: I'm still struggling. I was making progress for a while but now I'm not so sure. It's the *cha cha cha* of recovery. I had a migraine last night, so was drugged with a migraine hangover this morning. Our first group today was music therapy and I completely fell apart. The therapist had a basket of percussion instruments, all the things we'd give the kids in band back when I was teaching, like claves, maracas, clackers, tambourines etc. I was overwhelmed with grief. Which is ridiculous, given I chose to walk away from music and I know it was the right decision. I was so upset, I had to leave group. Then they drugged me and put me to bed. I had a good sob and hope I can finally put that grief behind me. I felt really flat for the rest of the day, then had another meltdown at dinner which is so humiliating. I saw how huge the meal was, and how unappetising, knowing how much difficulty I've been having getting food to go through the empty lap band. So, I sat and stared, and the gentle nurse kept encouraging me, but I couldn't do it. I left it all. Had to have the supplement instead. I'm hoping after the past few days of struggling, I can get my shit together and pull my socks up and get on with this recovery business. I don't know how to effectively deal with anxiety and that has to become an integral part of this process. I find the discouragement of forming friendships with other patients extremely disturbing and very difficult. It goes against the very essence of my being to see someone struggling and upset and not react or respond in some capacity. I understand the logic, but I hate it.

Day Twenty-Eight: I learned today my mother was right about one thing; absence truly does make the heart grow fonder. I've been incarcerated for four weeks, and yesterday was the first time I've seen Mick since I arrived. We've had two whole days together and have a therapy session tomorrow before he flies home. We've never been apart for four weeks, and it really is quite a stretch of time. Particularly as I'm in an unfamiliar, difficult place, and I know he struggles emotionally when I'm not there. As I'm now elevated to phase two, I can go out over one meal, twice a week. So, we left the clinic from 10:15 a.m. to 3:15 p.m. yesterday and today—five whole hours of normality. He was given instructions on when and how much I should eat and the post-meal supervision rules, then we headed back to his hotel and tried to forget all about the separation and just enjoy time together. After the obligatory conjugal relations were done and dusted, we ordered room service, then indulged in my most anticipated activity of the weekend. He dyed my hair. My hairdresser sent a little box with half a dozen tubes of colour and some hydrogen peroxide, plus a mixing bowl and comb. Mick meticulously measured ten grams of this and twenty grams of that onto the scales until the perfect paste was formed. We followed the instructions, and an hour later—leaving a blood bath in the hotel bathroom—my hair was back to its proper colour, no regrowth shining through. Today we headed out for a lovely lunch, a beautiful stroll along the riverside, and then, quite by happy accident, we discovered a shopping mall. The rest of the day we spent at the clinic, mostly snuggled up and snoozing as I'm so damn tired all the time. It was lovely spending so much time together. Which isn't a sentence I've said out loud—or even thought—for a long time. I'll be sad to farewell him tomorrow. While I find myself feeling wobbly from time to time, I'm also totally committed to recovery. Which looks to be a combination of creating new habits—sticking with them long enough that they are comfortable and familiar—and learning to effectively manage depression and anxiety. Plus, somehow (and this is the big unknown) finding a way to accept my body and value myself. And it has to come from me. This is the biggest obstacle. But I can only climb one mountain at a time.

Day Thirty-Two: Had ward round today; I'm moved up to phase three. Now I can go out three times per week. Also discussed my continuing issues with anxiety. I've been moved to a different non-optional med three times per day as part of my normal meds. My psychiatrist asked me to write a list of all the things I worry about. When I said everything, he said, "Put that at the top of the list." I've filled seven pages so far. No sign of a discharge date as he's waiting for me to feel confident about managing my eating—without regressing to the binge-purge-restrict cycle. Sheree waltzed in this afternoon, her usual vibrant ball of energiser bunny, filled with too many thoughts to get them all out at once. It was so gorgeous to see her; I've missed her! I even have special leave to go out for six hours with her on Sunday—to go to church, which will be an interesting experience. I've only ever attended church for weddings and funerals—usually as a performer. I did take away one brief comment from her today, and that's my inclination to focus on the negative. I'm not sure when this happened; most of my life, I was the eternal optimist. But somewhere along the way, that was beaten out of me. I'm not sure if this is good or bad as I've read studies that say optimists are frequently more disappointed than pessimists. But I know some time over the last decade, I became very protective of myself—anticipating the worst but hoping for the best. When the worst does happen, it somehow seems easier to deal with. One of the lovely *Doctor Who's* did once say (and I paraphrase): *What's the point of worrying? You just experience the problem twice.* I think my eternal worrying comes from wanting to map out a solution for an as-of-yet, non-existent problem. But nonetheless, her comment left me wondering how and when I changed. And should I change back? And if so, how?

Day Thirty-Three: I showed my seven pages of *things Simone worries about* to the psychiatrist this morning. He asked me to read out the list, clarified things needing more information, and validated they are all reasonable worries, and I have a lot on my plate. The trick is to learn to manage the worry. He wants me to download a mindfulness app again and give that a try. I suck at mindfulness. This evening, I went to dinner with Sheree and her husband. I even sat in a car for ten minutes which I haven't done since I arrived thirty-three days ago. It was so normal. Traffic and parking and ordering food and eating it and having a glass of wine (on top of my meds) and having conversation and just being normal. It eased some of my fears about going home. In group today, I talked about how I'm both really keen and really scared to go home. Keen, because this isn't life; I have no control or purpose or strong, meaningful connections, or freedom here. I can't sleep in, charge my devices by myself, snuggle my cat, go for coffee, see my friends, drive my car, watch Netflix, drink from a glass, or go bushwalking in Tasmania's wilderness. But I'm also scared, because I've come so far, and I don't want to slip back. I'm eating food (constantly), maintaining a stable weight, supported twenty-four/seven, surrounded by people who understand, and I have no responsibilities. So, it's safe—protecting me from the eating disorder—but it's also cutting me off from having a meaningful life. There was discussion—and consensus—on the fact that there will come a time when I'll know I've learned all I can and be ready to go out into the real world and practice trusting myself. The only way to know how I'll go at home is to go home. My psychiatrist is looking for confirmation from me that I'm feeling confident that I can be trusted. I'm nearly there. Not 100 per cent—but nearly. When I'm on leave, I'm pulled into doing the wrong thing, but I keep reminding myself *that was the old me.* The new me is practising new ways.

Day Thirty-Seven: Today I shed a thousand tears. And when they dried, I shed a thousand more. I woke to news a friend of twenty-two years died suddenly in her sleep. Our friendship is hard to quantify; Linda lived in Florida in the US, and I live in Tasmania, Australia. Far, far away from each other. Yet for twenty-two years, we communicated—with a group of around forty women—almost daily. Our initial common bond was pregnancy and a due date of August 1996. But before long, we discussed everything—birth and death, love and loss, sex, drugs, and rock 'n roll. Friendships aren't formed solely in close proximity, but through mutual love, respect, and understanding. Today, Linda's three sons begin life with no living parent. While she's reunited with her soul mate, three young men are left reeling with an unexpected and tragic loss. In 2010, I had the great privilege of meeting Linda and a dozen of the other mums. I felt an instant kinship as we shared the highs and lows of raising three boys with high intelligence and wills of iron. We laughed and cried and hugged and an amazing friendship from afar was consolidated in the flesh. I'm shocked beyond words that such a vibrant, passionate woman has gone so quickly and far too soon. I'll miss her comments on my blog. I'll miss her wisdom in our group. I mourn that we only met once in real life. I want to go home now—I'm ready—and I want a set date. Today is the first day I've ever experienced grief and loss and not been permitted to be hugged or consoled by anyone. I could have done with a hug. I want to go home.

Day Thirty-Eight: Today is the beginning of the end. And this auspicious ending will soon lead to the end of the beginning. I had my ward round today, and it was promptly suggested that I might like to move onto the pre-discharge phase. Yes, please! This means I have leave seven days per week. Monday-Friday 2-8 p.m. and weekends 8:30 a.m.-7:30 p.m. It's an adjustment phase to experience a bit of real life. Most patients live close by, but I don't. I'll have to go shopping or to the theatre instead. It allows me to see how I cope when I'm left in charge of myself for long periods of time. I'm not worried about eliminating thoughts; I just want to feel confident that I'll have no compulsive urges to follow through with disordered behaviours. Only time will tell, but at this point, I'm starting to feel more confident. I also have a discharge date two weeks from today, two weeks to hone my newly learned behaviours and work through issues or obstacles that arise. My anticipated six-week stay lasting longer than expected, the doctors wanted me to be ready. My flight's booked. Mick will fly over the Sunday before I leave, so he can meet with the family therapist and dietitian and go home with as much information as possible to support me as I adjust back to real life. I've made appointments with my dietitian, psychologist, and a psychiatrist when I return. I want to discuss a tweaking of my menu plan before I'm discharged. I can't change things here as the programme is for all of us—not just my unique set of issues. But the dietitian agreed to talk about modifying the plan I use at home.

Day Forty-Two: Today is the forty-second day of my incarceration and my fifty-second birthday. Six weeks ago, when it dawned on me that I would be spending my birthday in a psychiatric hospital, I felt really dreary. I celebrate so few of my birthdays, and this year, I wanted to get together with friends and celebrate properly. Instead, I was alone. I had the most wonderful day. The girls in the clinic sang happy birthday at breakfast (not something I'm generally comfortable with). I went to the city early and waited for Koko Black to open so I could have morning tea at one of my favourite places in Melbourne. An artisan chocolate shop. Ironically, I wasn't in the mood for chocolate, so had house-made crumpets with fresh butter and raspberry jam with cacao nibs. Delicious. I pottered around in Myer until lunchtime, then went back to Koko Black. They do a delightful goat cheese and caramelised onion toasted sandwich as well as the usual chocolate delights. Perfect. I purchased chocolates to have for afternoon tea, then headed to the theatre to watch *Beautiful: The Carole King Musical*. It was sublime, and I was only four rows from the front. I could see and hear perfectly. I had just enough time to drop into the cinema and watch *I, Tonya*. Amazing film and Margot Robbie is fabulous. Mick sent a message telling me to Facetime him ASAP. I immediately panicked, but he had all four boys plus my dad—and cat— over for dinner, so I chatted to them all while they wished me a happy birthday. I headed back to the clinic, grabbing a caesar salad for dinner first. No problems eating, and back with three minutes to spare. While technically I celebrated my birthday alone, I did lots of things I adore and felt very loved with all the calls and messages. Turning fifty-two isn't all that bad. While I'm a lot older than I used to be, it's fair to say I'm potentially a lot younger than I'm going to be. It was a great day, and for that, I'm very thankful.

Day forty-four: Today, I've crashed emotionally. I'm not sure if it's fear rearing its ugly head as I near the discharge date, or there are other things going on, but let's just say it's a good thing I didn't take leave from the clinic as leaping in front of a train seemed an attractive option. I don't believe I would do it, but it's a nice daydream. I'm overly tired and slept a lot between meals and groups—to the point where the trainee nurse let me know I was late for every meal. It's difficult with all the new girls on the unit and their level of distress. I don't feel compelled to do anything. The nurses sit with them and talk through stuff (plus it's none of my business), but I feel emotions so strongly. Even other people's. It's like a change in the air I'm breathing, and I inhale all their feelings and distress. I can't not do it, because I have to breathe the air. I feel it. So, today was hard. As is my way, I downloaded a playlist of miserable songs to feed the misery. I soak it in, accept it, feel it, write about it, go to sleep, and awake to a new day. I'm hoping that's what will happen at any rate. I haven't felt this low for weeks. I'm still gaining confidence with the eating stuff. Going home's scary, but that's par for the course. The only way through, is through. Next week, I'll pack up hospital life and head back to real life—hoping for the best.

Day Forty-Eight: I don't even know what to think, say, or write. I planned my day as carefully as possible to stay safe—safe from eating disorder behaviours, suicidal thoughts, and self-harm opportunities. And for the most part, I did well. Had my legs waxed, then a manicure and pedicure (luxuries I never do at home, so I'm calling it self-care and a way to fill in two hours with no harmful thoughts). Had morning tea on the way to the appointment, then straight to a café I know well. Felt safe. Back to the clinic until dinner time. Played a mindless word game on my phone all afternoon and napped. Went out for dinner, reassuring my nurse I'd walk straight to the restaurant I know (where it's easy to eat safe food) and walk straight back. She checked and said, "Are you sure you're safe?" I said I'd be fine—walk there, eat, walk back. Facetimed Sheree on the way there. Chatted to Kirsten. Had a lovely meal. Spied a knife that came with my meal and couldn't resist. It wasn't sharp, so not a huge amount of damage done. Just compulsive thoughts I can't stop. I left as soon as possible and walked straight back to the clinic. Found a piece of broken glass on the ground and scratched away for the fifteen-minute walk. Again, not much damage, but if I'd had the option to carve my arms up, I would. I've chatted to the nurse, and she's bandaged my arm. Now I have to be supervised in the common area, because I can't honestly guarantee I won't look for something else. I don't know why the overwhelming urges are back. I hadn't self-harmed since October. And that was a single incident after a couple of months. When I first came here, I scratched my hands, so they upped my medications. I'm not sure what's worse—self-harm or my eating disorder—if I have to choose between the two. Which is how it always feels. I know that's not the answer, but as I become more accepting of letting the eating disorder go and making plans for recovery at home, the urge to self-harm escalates. I can't see a doctor or registrar until Monday. I have my leave cancelled until I've seen a doctor which isn't enormously convenient but completely understandable. I'm disappointed and frustrated at a backward step just as I'm ready to discharge. I'm struggling to turn it around. The only solution feels like ensuring I'm never left alone. Which isn't a realistic long-term strategy.

Day Forty-Nine: Three sleeps to go. Today was a good day. No angst. No white-knuckling. No issues. Mick arrived bearing roses, and while I wasn't allowed to leave the building, we spent a lovely couple of hours curled up on my bed chatting and snoozing. He has a couple of odd heart conditions, so it's fascinating to lie on his chest and listen to the weird erratic patterns. Apparently normal for him—hasn't killed him in fifty-six years, so fingers crossed it won't any time soon. I'll be seeing my psychiatrist in the morning and will beg to be allowed back on leave. Escorted leave is fine. I just don't want to spend my last days couped up in a tiny room. Plus, we need to buy another suitcase, and I don't trust Mick to buy the right one. Over the next two days, we have appointments with the dietitian and family therapist to work out plans and supports that need to be in place when I get home. He'll do anything he can to help, but he isn't instinctive; he needs instructions. And I'm not the right person to set the guidelines as I can never tell whether I'm being led by reason or insanity. I'm feeling positive and hopeful about managing recovery when I get home, but worried about transference to self-harm. I haven't conquered anxiety and it needs to become a priority. I need pharmacological support for now. The urges were mild today, but I was medicated, stuck in the clinic, and had company most of the day. I'm also temporarily playing a mindless word game as it's a numbing distraction that seems less harmful but obviously isn't dealing with the key issue.

I guess it's something to work on with my psychologist at home.

BELIEVE ME

Day Fifty-Five: I'm home but still journaling for now. When urges to do anything maladaptive crop up (eating disorder, self-harm, *Candy Crush*, online shopping, name your problem), I'm encouraged to journal. My writing mentor would say *write into it*. So here I am, writing into it. I have no understanding of this sudden desire to binge. Mostly, I've desired to starve since I returned home from the clinic. I haven't. I've been extremely compliant and followed my meal plan. I keep eating when I'm full, because apparently, it takes a lot longer for my body to recognise natural hunger signals. I can't trust my body. I can't trust my head. I have to trust the professionals who worked with me to develop an eating plan specific to my needs upon returning home. This afternoon, I spent four hours with my hairdresser—a delightful way to spend a Saturday afternoon. It has been many moons since my hair has had the full loving care of my expert hairdresser. I had a cup of tea and a biscuit while I was there. Then came home and had two more biscuits. I don't know if I've had two afternoon teas or two halves of one afternoon tea. The confusion is messing with my head. Or perhaps it's the taste of Tim Tams. One is too many, and a hundred is never enough. Yet I've been cautioned not to avoid trigger foods as I'll remain in a permanent eating disorder mindset. So, I have a large snack box filled to the brim with every type of snack from my menu plan, all carefully portioned out into a snack-size serving. And twice a day, I choose a snack and have a piece of fruit with it. I'm hoping during these early uncomfortable days, I can retrain my brain to accept all food—not good versus bad. But just food. A daily diet of regularly feeding my body with a balance of nutrients. And no such thing as bad or off limits or foods that require punishment after eating. Apparently, this is how people with a healthy relationship with food behave. It's clear that I've never had a healthy relationship with food. After almost eight weeks of intensive recovery, I've been told on so many occasions that it's possible for this to happen. It takes time, courage, and persistence. But most of all, hope and belief. I have an enormous amount of belief and trust in the team of support people around—friends, family, and the professionals at home and the clinic. I also have a little bunny called Hope wearing a key necklace engraved with *hope*. When I go to bed each night, I find the bunny and say, *I have Hope*, and the words are becoming believable.

Day Fifty-Six: This is my final journal entry regarding my inpatient stay. I ended up staying fifty-two days in an intensive, militaristic, hard-line, no-messing-about, eating disorder programme, in a large psychiatric hospital. There were between ten and eighteen of us in the EDP at any one time. Most of the girls were twenty-ish, but there was another lady my age and one or two in their thirties and forties coming and going. At no point were we ever allowed to discuss our own particular eating disorder diagnosis, but to my non-expert eye, it would appear at least three-quarters of the girls were anorexic. I believe some were bulimic and some moved backwards and forwards from one to the other, as is so common in the eating disorder world. When I look at my journals, I realise how tough it was. It got easier; familiarity will do that. I learned a lot, and I'm so glad I had the opportunity to go. It wasn't fun. I didn't enjoy it. It wasn't the holiday a lot of people who don't know me well assumed I was on. I was apparently malnourished on arrival. They did regular blood tests, and I'm much better nourished now. Eating six meals per day will do that, especially if they've been tailored to my specific needs by a team of dietitians. While many of the rules were harsh and unrelenting, the staff were (mostly) amazing. I've now had two (voluntary) stays in psychiatric hospitals and learned mental health nurses are awesome. They're great at listening, drawing things out, getting to the heart of the matter, then finding perspective and forgiveness. My psychiatrist and his registrar were also great. Daily routine involved six very structured, specific, timed meals, followed by post-meal supervision. Eating and supervision took six and a quarter hours per day. We had a one-hour therapy session mornings and afternoons Monday-Friday was psychology and art/music/movement therapy. One day a week, we'd go to a café for a hot milk drink and some cake, then once a month, there's a lunch somewhere like a burger place for a burger and soft drink or juice. Eating out is about overcoming fear of bad foods. There's much discussion of the fact that food is food—neither good nor bad. We're constantly challenged with snacks many eating disordered people fear as off-limits. In my fifty-two days (416 meals and snacks), I normalised eating patterns, became better nourished, started to accept food is neither good nor bad (more work to do in this area), was reassured to learn eating regularly caused no weight gain (my greatest fear), and discovered the root cause of a lot of my issues is high anxiety buried for fifty years. This is something difficult to understand, problematic to accept, and a complete mystery to me as to how I can solve the conundrum. Working with my psychologist will be the most important tool, I guess, as staying sedated for every anxiety-inducing moment is not really feasible long-term. How have I gone my entire life and not known about anxiety? I always thought it was something my mother and sister had. But apparently I'm in the same boat. Time will tell if I sink or sail this boat. Probably one of the biggest gains of my stay was losing the desire to purge. I have zero interest in purging, but due to the lap band, it remains an issue. I vacillate between wanting to binge or restrict but have succumbed to neither. When wanting to restrict, I follow my meal plan (alarms go off on my phone six times a day) and eat anyway. I've had little desire to binge, but when it's come along, I've used past strategies like distractions and urge surfing, and they were successful. Self-harm is a constant desire but again, so far, I resist. I'm also conscious of the fact that right now I'm in a fairly stressless environment and have a lot of support and eyes on me. It's easier to do the right thing when things are going right. The strength of my recovery and progress will be best measured when life's next curveball is hurled my way. We all get them, and I'd be awfully naive to think life will be a bed of roses from now on. The more habitual good habits become, the easier it is to safely navigate stormy waters when they head my way; that's my new theory. I'm still exhausted all the time. You'd think all this nutrition would boost my energy, but not as of yet. My energy will return; I just have to give it time. I'm starting to pour what energy I have into writing. And I have a lot of planning to do for a three month trip to Europe which has been five years in the planning and is now only three months away. Life is full and busy, and I'm tentatively hopeful my intensive stay at the clinic will be a major turning point in my life. If I can get on top of fifty-plus years of disordered eating, then I can get on top of high anxiety. I have to believe that.

FOOD RULE 2,584

Eat three meals and three snacks per day.

THE GIRL WITH THE
EATING DISORDER

I identify as the girl with the eating disorder. I need a better identity. Friends often ask what they can do to help or support me. I'm usually flummoxed by this question. I have no idea how to help myself, so how can I provide information when I don't know? There are warning signs at the beginning of a slippery descent into the rabbit warren of mental unwellness—when the rabbit holes are a mere hop, skip, and a jump away. There are also things I do in a healthy headspace that are beneficial when my thoughts go haywire.

I've just returned from a most beautiful five days on Tasmania's Maria Island with Sheree. The island is uniquely stunning with its flora and fauna reserves, and historical ruins to explore. Physically, the trip was demanding. Normally I can walk forever without much problem, and love nothing better than climbing mountains to find a spectacular view to soak in, dangle my feet over a clifftop, and take a selfie of my shoelaces. But after seven weeks in a psychiatric facility where I was allowed no more exertion than walking to the dining table, my fitness has dropped. On our second day, we kayak down the west coast of the island, discovering long white sandy beaches and multi-coloured coves, and enjoying a very crisp swim before exploring on foot. We make the mistake of enjoying the pristine white beaches a little too long and have to kayak back to the penitentiary accommodation in windy, white caps, which is hard and

I'm trying not to go backwards in the water. Sheree is stronger, more experienced, and worried about my ability to get back. Just as she's yelling at me to keep digging in, a seal (apparently) leaps out of the water behind me, and she goes from worried to exhilarated in a flash. We make it back. I knew we would. It's one of those days where you're reminded to dig deep and keep going no matter what.

In the clinic, I learned to eat three meals and three snacks a day. Regular alarms are now set on my phone, and I've stopped living on cereal, and added proteins, vegetables, and healthy stuff that makes my body and brain function. I follow the three/five rule my dietitian set; every meal needs representatives from three of the five food groups in the Australian Dietary Guidelines. Even on Maria Island, I follow through with the plan. Sheree reminds me I must eat; it's the whole reason for the last couple of torturous months.

If I stop eating properly—skip breakfast, eat only when people see me, binge in the middle of the night, only eat cereal, don't drink water, completely restrict, or go into food refusal (I'm in a pretty bad headspace by then)—then my slippery descent has begun. But it always starts with that first step—skipping breakfast. And that decision comes from the most innocuous of reasons, a throw-away comment from someone, an unflattering photo, people sharing their weight on Facebook, my wedding ring feeling tight. It takes very little reason for the eating disorder voice to get all puffed up with self-importance and shout down the new voice I unearthed in the clinic.

At the end of our long day of weepy, seal-inspired, exhausting kayaking, I stare at dinner in tears and Sheree turns into nurse mode, insisting I get through it. Not with the strict time frames from the clinic, but with a firm insistence that she cooked food, and I've just spent all that time in the clinic, and there's no backing out now. She's tired too. I eat my dinner.

The next day, we cycle to the island's sandy isthmus. For Sheree, cycling is fine. For me, it's unnaturally terrifying. I haven't ridden a bike since I was fourteen years old. While some of the tracks are rocky, for the most part, they're good paths with plenty of flat and downhill sections. I'm still unnaturally terrified and can only put it down to high anxiety; it's not long since I left the clinic. By the end of the day, I finally start to settle and feel less nervous.

There's the old saying, you never forget how to ride a bike, and I guess that's true, because I didn't fall off. But you lose your nerve. My go-to distress tolerance behaviour is self-harm—scratching or tearing at my hands and feet, using implements when things go pear-shaped, suicidal ideation whenever I'm left on my own. It's my way of coping with anxiety—the instant numbing effect.

My inpatient stays and eternally patient psychologist have taught me some distress tolerance skills and the easiest one that comes to mind is always grounding—using my five senses to ground in the here and now. As we ride past the stands of eucalypts and myriad wandering wombats, I press my feet firmly onto the pedals. I try to sense everything touching my body—the firmness of my sports bra, sweaty hands on the handlebars, the uncomfortable strap from the bike helmet. I listen for the sound of the wind as it whooshes past my ears, the kookaburras and cockatoos in the trees, the waves lapping at the shore, all the sounds of nature we've come to soak up. I can smell the gum trees and taste the salty sea in the air. I repeat the process and breathe. Slowly. A mindfulness practise we've been taught. A mindfulness practise I've actually remembered. And it works. It helps. My anxiety about riding a bike around a mountainous sandy island, using long-forgotten muscles, keeping up with a strong, fit energiser bunny, starts to abate. By then it's almost dark.

After two physically taxing days on my heavily drugged and sedentary body, we sleep in, then climb a mountain. Walking is my comfort zone. I love it. I know moving my body is good for mental health. Not just going to the gym for an hour, but getting out and about every day, walking in nature, doing housework. Anything other than sitting on my butt feeling sorry for myself and wondering how long it takes to develop bedsores. Sometimes it's a drag and the voices in my head fight, but the rewards are worth it. We arrive at the top of Bishop and Clerk to spectacular views across the Freycinet National Park. Along the way, we pass bottlebrush and native orchids, echidnas, eastern grey kangaroos, and Cape Barren geese. We admire the rugged cliffs, big buttongrass moors, gentle pine forest walks, and we scramble over rocky scree before reaching the summit. Dangling my feet over the edge of the cliff, enjoying our packed lunch on the summit with the brisk wind messing up my hair as I gaze across the turquoise waters is my reward for surviving nearly two months in the clinic.

Despite exhaustion and teary days, progress from the clinic continues. Mick is supportive and checks my meals. I'm in contact with my professional team, and if I stuff up, I reach out and let someone know rather than wallow in shame. Sheree and Kirsten check in on me most days.

I've been doing this recovery gig a long time and keep asking my psychologist why the hell it's taking me this long to get my shit together, but apparently, patience is key, and everything will happen in its own time. Perhaps this is my time. Day to day life keeps on keeping on. I'm no longer in the paid workforce, but I'm perpetually busy with urgent demands that are as varied and fickle as a weather report.

I was stuck in traffic last week, without access to Bluetooth—a decidedly first-world problem. I turn on the radio. As fate would have it, the first station it landed on was a Christian station. I was curious about Sheree's faith and actually didn't realise there were Christian radio stations. Who knew? I had nothing else to do so tuned in to listen.

The traffic is busy, Hobart city experiencing its peak minutes as happens each morning, so there's plenty of slow time to tune in and listen. Frustratingly, the radio station isn't local, and the frequency is close to another station—determined to ruin my concentration by cutting in and out. As I drive along, trying to listen to my God station, I realise this is the story of my life.

Like you, I have a voice of wisdom, reason, logic, common sense, knowing, intuition, God—whatever resonates with your personal belief system—but for the vast majority of my life, there's another frequency butting in and drowning out the word I want (and need) to hear. Sometimes the noise of the unwanted station drowns the other out completely; I know it's there, but it can't be heard. Sometimes the station appears clear as crystal. Then it goes again.

When the radio station tunes in nicely, there's a sense of peace and acceptance—and enjoyment that the voice I want to hear is coming through loud and clear. The rest of the time, there's utter discord, and the stress becomes overwhelming. The temptation to let go of searching for that disappearing frequency is really strong; it's far easier to tune into the intrusion as it becomes stronger and clearer and to give up on the station I want and go with the one that's easy and comfortable.

This is the voice of insanity.

Christian friends call it the enemy. I call it the eating disorder voice - I don't know where it comes from as I've listened to it prattling away for half a century and it's only quite recently I even noticed another voice hidden in the background.

Tuning in to the voice of God is no mean feat. What does that even mean? Any one of us can talk to ourselves to the point where anything is acceptable and logical, but that's the deceptive voice. To muddle through a decision and come to a real knowing of its rightness requires not just self-knowing but external validation that your thought processes aren't concocting good excuses to do whatever it is you probably shouldn't do.

I'm not schizophrenic, and for that, I'm grateful. I have enough problems, and schizophrenia would be a biggie. But I do have long diatribes with myself that almost always end up leading to some kind of ineffective, destructive behaviour. Naturally, I spend a lot of time wondering why I'm such an idiot, but my radio experience, of two competing stations drifting in and out making it impossible to concentrate on the preferred station, gave me the insight to realise there's a lot of external noise inside my head. Finding recovery—especially long term recovery—is going to be completely dependent on tuning in to both voices, so I can gradually turn the wise voice up and the fearful voice down.

In the weeks and months following my return from the clinic, for the most part, life's okay. I eat my scheduled meals. Kirsten and I catch up for weekly talks and walks. Sheree and I start filming for her online business. Mick and I plan our big trip. I have endless appointments, and I write.

Picturing a future is difficult, but the more I try, the easier it gets. All those years lost in fantasy worlds of my beloved books aren't helping. Imagining a future as a professional ballet dancer isn't productive. Imagining a future where my book is published, I have a job, travel and spend time with friends and family—that has potential.

I've inadvertently built myself a new identity around mental health—or lack thereof—and part of my recovery is redefining a new me. It's hard to picture that I was once a different person altogether. When I cracked apart, all these problems started. Prior to that, I was just a normal person, blissfully unaware of issues simmering away which I'd numbed into non-existence in a most spectacular manner. Sometimes, I yearn for that ignorant girl.

Once I was a musician, student, chorister, administrator, mother, teacher, wife, daughter, friend. Now I have mental health problems. Now I'm the girl with the eating disorder.

THE BLANK SPOT

M y toes are pointing at a blank spot. A blank spot where my scales have sat since we renovated the bathroom eighteen years ago.

For as long as I can remember, I weighed myself first thing every morning, day in, and day out. Like clockwork. A special, comforting routine. I'd climb out of bed, empty bladder, strip naked, stare at the fateful numbers.

And for as long as I can remember, I have known this is a terrible thing to do. When the numbers go up, I panic and make stupid decisions about my eating. When the numbers go down, I fear they'll go back up, then I panic and make stupid decisions about my eating. There's no win. There's no time when I look at the numbers and think, *Awesome!* There are definitely times when I look back and wish I'd appreciated numbers, but I never appreciate them at the time. They're always a stepping-stone to a magical place that doesn't exist. Skinny equals happy-land.

I've finished an online bulimia recovery course and made a commitment to drop from daily to weekly weighing. I couldn't cope with the thought of getting rid of them completely, but over time, contemplated the thought of not weighing myself daily. Many tiny baby steps were all I could ask for. So, I dropped to weighing every seven-ten days.

This morning, I weighed in. Fateful number was okay. Not up or down, but I'm still not happy with it. I jumped online and caught up on recovery banter and noticed a lot of discussion about scales. There was some tough love tossed around, in a beautiful, empathetic manner, but it was still no bullshit, just tough love. And while I wasn't the original poster of the scales question, everything related to me completely.

I can't be dragged over the finish line.

I can't be forced to use the tools.

Nobody can do the work for me.

I already know what to do.

I need to get rid of the fucking scales.

I'll never feel good about getting rid of them.

Why do I want to weigh myself?

What do I hope to gain?

While I had the strength to do so, I sent Mick a message asking him to hide them away when he got home from work. I could have taken them outside and ceremoniously smashed them to bits, but that seems very wasteful for expensive scales and unfair on the rest of the family who use them from time to time—usually to weigh luggage.

I felt a lot of angst all day and weighed myself again at lunchtime, just for old time's sake. When I got home, the scales were gone. A big empty space on my white-tiled bathroom floor, right where they used to sit. No more weighing.

Kirsten said she's proud of me. I don't feel pride. I just feel angst. How will I know if I'm getting fatter? How will I know if I'm not? What will my new morning routine look like? How will I know what to wear each day? How will I know how much to eat each day?

But I also know this was a really good decision that I'll become more comfortable with over time. Change is meant to be uncomfortable. I hear that again and again. This is hugely uncomfortable, and I've roped Mick into it, so I don't just unhide them from myself or go buy a new set tomorrow. The longer I go not weighing, the more normal it should become. Theoretically. I guess answers to the questions above will become clear over time.

Throwing away the scales is the end of a monumental era for me. But more than that, I think it powerfully indicates I've found the right path and started moving forward. I've traversed many roads, and none have led to anywhere near this kind of improvement; for me, they were the wrong road. Or perhaps little back roads bringing me to the highway. Everything I'm doing now is heading in the right direction.

UP, UP, & AWAY

A lifetime in the dreaming. Five years in the planning. Three months in the doing. Europe 2018, here we come.

But first, I have—both literally and figuratively—been swamped. And as it so happens, when I'm swamped, I unravel. Again.

Our house flooded in May. It's a bit of a bummer really. Accompanied by angst and stress. We're fortunate in many (most) ways; the floors are ruined, but there's no structural damage, and we have good insurance to cover most of the repairs. But getting flooded is a pain in the ass. Aside from the extra expenses insurance won't cover, it's a week of packing up most of the house (by myself) to store in the shed and weeks of living without floor coverings while listening to the gentle roar of three industrial fans. It's also forced us into unplanned, premature, costly renovations. I know in six months' time, this will be history, and I'll have lovely new floors and plasterwork, but right now the stress has got to me, and my recovery isn't solid enough to avert relapse. So, relapse I have.

My friendship with Sheree is under huge strain, with all the stress of filming for her online fitness business. I spend a lot more time with Sheree than my other close friends as we're both relatively free during the day, a by-product of me no longer being in the paid workforce. In comparison to the longevity and comfort I have with The Girls, Emma and Kerry, my friendship with Sheree is new and volatile—not yet familiar enough to coast through the wobbles of familiarity. I fear I'll lose her every time I stuff up. I've inadvertently become a part of the business team—impromptu videographer, editor, communications and media expert, personal assistant. I believe passionately in Sheree's ability to transform women's lives. But mixing work and friendship doesn't always run smoothly. I feel ashamed at the volatility and tell nobody.

When it rains, it pours. Again, quite literally in this case. Mick has ventricular tachycardia and the powers-that-be are insistent he has radiofrequency ablation—aka surgery—before our flights to London. Which are twenty-six days away. Count them. Twenty-six days until we fly to London. He has to have heart surgery before then. In Melbourne, because it can't be done in Tasmania. Fuck. The house is underwater. It's raining. It's pouring. My coping mechanisms have washed down the drain.

When I first left the eating disorder clinic seventy-eight days ago, I ate (reluctantly) on a tight schedule. A little alarm on my watch taps me on the wrist five times a day, and it's my responsibility to eat the appropriate meal at the appropriate time. But I'm the first to admit after fifty-plus years of disordered eating, being responsible doesn't come naturally. In fact, it goes against every instinct I have, and I have to fight really hard to comply. And I mean really hard.

When life's tough, and stress overwhelms, fighting eating disorder thoughts takes more than I have. Consequently, over the past month, I've whittled away at routines and started to add or subtract meals and succumb to the desire for a lot less nutrition. It took just one unexpected comment about my weight to make me stop eating altogether. The desire to never eat again is tantalising and calls to me like a seductive siren from the sea. It's only with the support of my psychologist, and by finding the courage and strength to talk things through with Mick, Kirsten, and Sheree, that I can stop relapse in its tracks.

When you're a middle-aged woman, it's kind of expected you can feed yourself. But, you know what? I can't. If left to my own devices, I go astray. I need to be told what to eat and when. I need to be told when *not* to eat. I need to be treated like a child. I don't need to be asked if I'd like something to eat; the answer is always no. I didn't learn healthy behaviours as a child, so it seems I have to learn them now. And I can't learn them in seventy-eight days. Intellectually, I know the theory, but life isn't an intellectual exercise. It's emotional and habitual and real. And when reality becomes highly emotive, the oldest habits are the first to rise. I can't stay in a child-like state, but apparently, I have to start there.

I have ingrained one good habit over the past two years—talk about it and reach out. To my psychologist, my husband, and my friends. And to you—whoever you may be. Sharing stops me in my tracks and redirects me to the path I'm meant to be on.

I know those who've never suffered the shame of an eating disorder are unlikely to ever fully understand the depths of depravity and despair we hide. I also know coming out of hiding makes me accountable and steers me back on track. I want recovery so incredibly badly. But I want to run and hide from emotional distress even more. Old habits die hard, but kill them I will. It won't happen in seventy-eight days. It probably won't happen in a year. But it will happen. Through all sorts of therapies and chats with the wickedly wise and wonderful people who support me during various times of crises, I'm always reminded that intense feelings pass. No matter how distressed I am, hanging in there and waiting for the wash of emotions to fade will see me through the other side. There are so many clichés: urge surfing, riding the wave, sit with the emotions, this too shall pass. And they're true. Each and every one of them. Unfortunately, eating disorder recovery is a slow, painful process.

This time last week, my frantic levels of anxiety were receding. I had a sense of things finally coming together and falling into place. I dared to hope the dream might come true. This time two weeks ago, I was a mess. I'd cracked under pressure—again. Filled with suicidal ideation and a desperate need for sleep. I over-medicated twice—an overdose, I'm told. Although that wasn't my intention, and I required no medical intervention. But apparently, I could have accidentally died. I didn't care.

The trouble with cracking wide open and falling apart is cracks take a long time to heal. And they're fragile. When stress comes along, logic doesn't help. The anxiety is overwhelming, and sometimes the chaos so complete, there are no thoughts. Just all-consuming dread and fear. And the hardest thing is knowing it doesn't make sense. Of course, this too shall pass, but fear consumes, and acceptance is a distant concept.

That was two weeks ago. Now it too has passed. I surfed the urges (mostly), rode the emotional tidal waves, and made it here. To London. To the beginning of the holiday we've planned for five years.

I sobbed for most of the four-hour flight from Melbourne to Perth— mostly with waves of pain cascading through my back. But partly letting go of the emotional build-up to our departure, filled with the angst of travel plans (not fun), post-flood renovations (also unfun), and Mick's heart surgery. When the wheels lifted in Melbourne, it was all behind me.

London has been underwhelming. It was always our jumping-off point for the big adventure. Somewhere to recover from jet lag and begin the trip without too much stress. And it has done just that.

We've wandered around aimlessly each day, returning to our little haven to nurse various aches and pains. We've spectacularly discovered the worst food and coffee London has to offer. The skies are blue, the sun is shining, the sunset views from our bedroom window are truly spectacular. The United Kingdom is in the midst of an unbelievable heatwave, and accommodations are not equipped to cope. Iconic landmarks seem to know we're visiting and are clad in scaffolding or surrounded by workmen's barriers. Big Ben's little face peaks through a giant metallic condom.

Monday, we'll collect a car in Salisbury and the real adventure begins. Exploring the English countryside before heading to Jordan, Turkey, Sarajevo, Budapest, Krakow, Berlin, Berbiguières in the South of France, then Paris, where Mick will fly home and The Girls will fly over to share my last three weeks in Paris, Lucca, and Portugal, before we all head home.

But in the meantime, today I'll see an osteopath and sports massage therapist to sort the severe pain in my back and legs from the broken seat on the long-haul flight. Limping my way from London to Paris was never part of the plan. Nor was medicating myself into a state of oblivion. I'm hoping for miracles.

I feel calm. I know real life awaits at home, but for three months, I'm in a bubble of spoiled privilege. I want to soak up every moment—the best and the worst all rolling into one big adventure with tales to be told later on. After five years of planning, squirrelling away pennies and inheritances, and wondering if it will ever happen, we've made it. After five weeks of panic and stress and cracking apart at the seams yet again, we're here.

SPIRIT FIND ME

I 'm searching for something, and I don't know what it is. But I do know what it isn't. It isn't physical. Or psychological. It isn't health or wealth or happiness—although they're lovely and I'd like more, please. I'm not looking for religion; I need something far more personal.

The only word that makes sense to me is *spiritual*.

When I talk about God or religion or spirituality with my family, they ask, *why? What for?* And I don't know how to answer. I just know there's something in me that's become increasingly unsettled in recent years. Most profoundly in the year my psychological health unceremoniously splattered on the floor like an egg with no shell. Everything always comes back to 2015. From there, everything changed. Sometimes worse. Sometimes better.

I have friends with strong faiths, and I'm envious of the comfort they find in knowing God. I wish it was easy to just believe. I've tried. I even googled *how to believe in God*. But it isn't that simple. I don't even know if that's what I'm looking for.

In Edinburgh (I love Edinburgh!), I saw a sign that said *Try praying. It's easier than you think. Free guide at trypraying.co.uk.* I was on the way to the airport for a long flight to Jordan with a midnight layover in Istanbul, so I figured it would give me something to do. And it was a cool looking sign with a good-looking fella on it. I downloaded the app and followed the instructions. Simple enough. Not too weird or preachy. And I practised the twelve-step principle of *take what I need and leave the rest*. Which seems like a good principle for almost anything in life. Throughout the rest of our travels, I maintained a daily practice of quiet prayer. I learned to say the word God without tripping over my feet—something I refused to do in all the Overeater's Anonymous meetings I attended in the past. I learned to genuinely reach out to something beyond myself. Who or what remains a mystery. I just know it isn't me.

In the past week, we've travelled through Jordan, visiting breathtaking historical and biblical sites and walking where ancient peoples once watched the violent birthplace of Christianity. It's an amazing country and an incredible experience. It's also searingly hot, not my favourite temperature. Despite the constant need to reapply deodorant and the indignity of collapsing from the heat on red soil in a white shirt at Petra, I've loved this country and been drawn to the religious histories of Judaism, Islam, and Christianity. So many commonalities yet politics most often plays on the differences.

Regardless of religious belief, the history is fascinating. The deep sense of spirituality within the biblical sites resonates with me. I find so much peace sitting alone in ancient churches, where countless men and women have sought solace. So much comfort walking where ancient peoples once trod to carry water to their homes or gathered food for their families. I've taken every opportunity to sit and linger in each church, wondering how Moses and John the Baptist felt in millennia past. Listening peacefully. Imagining the spirit and the prayer that has filled the walls over the centuries. Quietly listening for the voice of God. He's silent.

Today was the last of our tours, at The Baptism Site of Jesus Christ. Allegedly. Despite Mick's cynical view of the historical accuracy, it was the most touching experience I've had here. Literally. I stood in the Jordan River and doused myself in the cool, muddy water. It was 41°C in the shade and we walked a kilometre to get there, so I was grateful for cool water on my arms, face, and back while dangling my feet in the shallow river. There were a handful of tourists and a very serious armed guard nearby, with the blue and white tape separating Jordan from Israel a few meters away, but I felt very alone for those few moments. Cool and peaceful. I didn't hear the voice of God or feel a thunderbolt strike me, but it was incredibly special. I don't know why.

As always happens with tours, we had obligatory stops at the gift shop before and after walking to the holy sites. It was blessedly air-conditioned which was a relief, as the heat was making me nauseous. I bought a tiny wooden cross that I bathed in the river with me. I don't know why I want it. I'm not Christian, but I feel pulled towards the Abrahamic religions.

My little anxiety-relieving bunny now has a tiny wooden cross hanging next to his silver key inscribed with hope. He feels extra special. I still hug him every night and say *I have Hope*. Since leaving the clinic in March, it's been my mantra—*I have Hope*. When depression or anxiety drags me down, *I have Hope*. I'm still searching for something. I don't know what it is. But bathing my arms and legs in the Jordan River brings me one step closer.

I feel a change. Something has shifted within me. An acceptance.

I fell in love with Jordan and hope to return. We spent eleven nights here, exploring all the ancient, holy sites and meeting the most beautiful, kind people. From Jordan, we continue our travels another sixty-six days through eight more countries, exploring histories growing ever closer to modern-day. We return home $40,000 poorer. A financial burden from which we may never recover. I regret nothing. The money was found through inheritances, five years of savings and paying off travel expenses over twelve months. My fears of travelling with a grumpy, angry Mick were unfounded; he was fabulous. We become close once more and had an incredible once-in-a-lifetime experience. The one-way ticket to Guatemala I cancelled all those years ago, when we promised to travel together soon, now finally replaced with a European tour previously unimaginable.

In every single country, I visit churches. Sometimes I go to a service. Sometimes I sit and admire the centuries old architecture. In Budapest, we walk two hours in searing heat for a church service, and for the first time, I walk to the front and ask for healing prayers. I explore church services in foreign countries where nobody knows me, and I feel no pressure to return, so I can understand without judgment. There's judgment from Mick. If he could roll his eyes further back, they'd spin in his head. But me going to church is none of his business. This is my recovery. My journey.

And I've found God now.

Some people rejoice. Others wring their hands and wonder what the fuck happened. I neither know nor care.

My entire life has been spiritually bereft, and it turns out that hasn't been entirely beneficial for my mental health. I grew up without any type of faith, something for which I am, and will always be, very appreciative. Whatever beliefs I carry and develop from this point forward have been developed in adulthood and with full cognisance of all the pros and cons of taking on a spiritual belief housed within the confines of traditional religion. I have no past experiences to colour my beliefs—merely a four-year journey to find comfort and healing from my own mental struggles, something I've come to realise cannot be done without a spiritual grounding. For some, that's a higher power. Others seek answers in the universe, nature, or community, and many people find spirituality in God. I'm one of those people.

My astonishingly intelligent husband and children question how I believe in something without concrete proof. I want to. That's all I need. That's faith—believing in something for which there's no evidence. I believed in angels when I was a little girl. My grandmother said I can't believe in angels if I don't believe in God. Why not? Who makes the rules about what's acceptable or unacceptable in a personal faith? Not grandma—I'm quite certain of that.

I've learned loads of recovery tools for depression, anxiety, self-harm, and disordered eating. But for whatever reason, I'm still floundering more than four years down the track. I don't need more tools and tips, tricks and resources; I need belief in myself and in a future I can't picture. And that requires faith.

I don't like blind faith. Blind faith requires outsourcing—grounding spiritual or religious belief and practice in external forces. I'm not comfortable with that. My core moral values have been developed, honed, and consolidated over five decades. They won't suddenly backflip because I've found faith in God. I prefer a softer approach—looking for beauty, strength, and love in God, as many millions of people have found comfort and solace over generations.

Spiritual awareness is new and unfamiliar to me. I was raised to be pragmatic and practical. Useful and helpful. There was no room for emotional expression, and as someone with an abundance of emotion, this was problematic. My solution was pragmatic; don't feel anything and don't display emotion. Bury everything and get on with being useful.

As I began the slow decline into a complete unravelling, all those suppressed emotions started rising to the surface like a thousand beach balls I'd valiantly endeavoured to keep below the surface of the water. Eventually, it was impossible. That's when I started searching for answers.

Spending time looking outside myself to the greater mysteries of life and conversing with God (ensuring it's a two-way conversation) are cornerstones of my recovery. More often than not, I forget to even ask God to lend me his strength, wisdom, and grace. As time makes its inevitable march forward, I hope releasing control of all my burdens will become a more natural process. Faith in God is not a pre-requisite for spirituality, but I've come to believe those of us struggling with recovery from [name your issue] remain stuck until spiritual practice and acceptance is found. I've met highly spiritual atheists and spiritless Christians, so where we find the willingness to look outside ourselves is personal. For me, the search ended with a traditional faith in God—something for which I will not apologise.

THE HSP

One way or another, we all feel different, but some differences are too much, while others are celebrated. What's curious is that sensitivity is rarely considered a positive trait in twenty-first century living. Being sensitive is being different. It's inconvenient for others. Yet if more of the populace was highly attuned to the feelings of others, we'd live in a kinder world.

I'm a Highly Sensitive Person (HSP). It's a thing; go Google it. It's also a spectrum, and I'm way up the top. For those of us sitting high on the spectrum, life can be overwhelming. In addition to being acutely sensitive to sight, sound, touch, taste, and smell, HSPs are often empaths and introverts. Empaths because we feel and absorb the emotions bleeding from those around us no matter how they try to hide it. Introverts because refuge and recuperation from overwhelming sensory input can require time alone to regenerate the energy and will to face another day.

I personally score top marks in all three areas.

The eighty-eight days I travelled around Europe were an incredible gift, experience, and all sorts of other happy adjectives. But I was also rarely alone. As someone who requires alone time to recharge, it was overwhelming. Being cooped up in a hotel room day in day out with someone—even someone I know as intimately well as my husband or closest friends—wore me down.

While most of my travels were filled with wide-eyed wonder, contentment, gratitude, and peace, I also experienced increasing levels of anxiety as my inability to spend time alone to recharge my inner battery dragged me down faster and faster. Time with The Girls gave me more time alone, as we're not precious about doing things together, so sometimes they'd go out and I'd stay in. Having friends I've known for thirty years is a tremendous blessing as I'm not sure many others could manage my increasing levels of stress through Italy and Portugal, where I eventually stopped eating and Kirsten unceremoniously handed me a tub of yoghurt and a spoon and said, "Eat this," while I was awaiting a home visit from an English speaking Portuguese doctor. He prescribed anxiety medications and other scripts I'd run out of, gave me detailed instructions on how to get to the pharmacy, phoned ahead to order the medications, and charged an exorbitant amount of non-claimable euro for the privilege. It was worth every penny.

I hadn't slept for a week. I retrieved the medications. Slept. And loved Portugal.

Hypersensitivity is too much for most people; we're told to toughen up, be more resilient, don't take things so personally. Good advice if you want the personality of a slab of concrete—emotions buried six-feet under. Not particularly useful if you want to be a fully functioning adult in a complex world. Twelve-step meetings are full of hypersensitive souls lacking the tools to cope with the bombardment of sensory input around them.

While my anxiety diminished over the remainder of our trip, I became paranoid about the flight home—worried about the pain I'd experienced on the way over, fearful of my severe restless legs annoying the adjacent passenger (Kirsten and I were on the same flight but not seated together), jealous of Mick flying home first class with all our Frequent Flyer points, sad the trip was over, scared about what the future holds and my soon-to-be-burst bubble, stressed knowing I'd be awake for forty or so hours, terrified about managing food in a confined space and just generally anxious.

After our layover in Doha, I'm relieved to discover a spare seat between the other passenger and myself. I decide to take a few medications and increase my chance of being calm and relaxed on the way home. My new habit of borderline overdose is taking hold. I eat dinner, order a Baileys, and down a little concoction of twenty-six pills. Bit of this. Bit of that. I don't really remember anything much for the next few days, but Kirsten does. She was concerned. The air hostess was concerned. I assumed I slept, but apparently not. She thinks I took more tablets because I couldn't asleep. When we wandered around Sydney airport for a few hours, she said I seemed pretty normal. I don't remember being at Sydney airport. Or Hobart airport. I don't remember arriving home. I lost about forty-eight hours of my life.

It frightens and shames me, to be publicly off my face. Drug addict is not really my thing. But the desire to wipe myself out of existence and sink into a blessed sleep of nothingness for a few hours is sometimes overwhelming. Sleep is more elusive than unicorn feathers and dragon fur in my world, so when things become overwhelming, I've added a new way of numbing myself—borderline overdose. There's often talk in the world of addiction of transference—moving the focus of addiction from one substance to another. I don't seem to do that; I just collect more options, so I have more choices. My recovery tool bag is full of healthy ways to manage emotional distress, but I'm still hypersensitive, need time alone to recharge, and I'm deeply affected by the emotions of those around me.

I still live in fear that shit will hit the fan. I find it hard to let go of the fear someone will die, my kids will get into trouble, someone will become really ill, I'll lose my job, I'll be in a high-conflict situation, we'll have a financial disaster, my marriage will fail, or any one of the myriad stresses my hyped-up head comes up with. And I still hark back to the safety net of ineffective behaviours.

I know cutting isn't a great coping tool. In fact, it's an avoiding tool. It just defers the emotional turmoil and acceptance of the situation to a later date. Yet the thought of getting rid of the blades I've stashed everywhere sends my anxiety levels sky-high. To feel safe, they have to be with me at all times—which did make recent interstate flights slightly problematic.

My large stash of medications put away for just-in-case are challenging to let go, but now I dip into them from time to time, so the stash becomes smaller rather than larger and there'll come a point where it's no longer a lethal dose. That hidden cache makes me feel safe. At any time of my choosing, if emotional and psychological pain becomes too overwhelming to endure, I can opt out.

The safety nets I've relied on in my disordered eating are purging and restricting, as well as constant weighing. I've made intermittent progress, but most importantly, have started to believe perhaps recovery is a remote possibility. I ditched the weighing, but the thought of not purging and restricting is so foreign that I can barely comprehend it. And the thought of not engaging in those behaviours is severely anxiety-inducing.

The irony of hypersensitivity is a tendency to diminish, bury, or invalidate personal feelings and experiences to the detriment of self. I think the world needs us. An ever-shrinking global landscape needs people to see through the deception of carefully constructed facial expressions and the increasing prevalence of artfully manipulative political leaders. We need more folk to care for the humanity of spirit over the blind greed of material wealth and to work quietly in the shadows making this world a better place, simply because it's a beautiful thing to do—not for glory, accolades, or financial reward.

Today, I went to church. Not because I was asked to, but to find people who believe in God and Jesus and miracles. Who profess faith in a humble man who preached love, kindness, compassion, and goodness. Because I yearn to find more people like that in the world and in my spiritual quest. I think if Jesus walked the earth today, he'd be a highly sensitive, empathic introvert, acutely aware of the feelings of those around him. An expert reader of body language. And a man who took time alone to recharge his batteries as he communed with his Father.

FOOD RULE 4,181

Don't purge.

BYE BYE BAND

In 2012, I became the happy recipient of a gastric lap band. In 2019, I'm having it removed.

I'm petrified.

Not of the surgery itself. Surgery never bothers me, and this is a quick, easy procedure (if you're a surgeon). But the thought of going back to fully unrestricted eating is, quite frankly, terrifying. On numerous levels.

Prior to the lap band, I spent forty-six of my forty-six years obsessed with food—eating too much, feeling guilty, trying to eat less, failing, dieting, gaining weight, losing weight, gaining it back with a little bit extra. In tears and absolute desperation, I turned to my GP who sent me to the lap band surgeon. I had the surgery four days later.

From that point, weight peeled away quite consistently. But the flip side of that happy coin was the rapid expansion of my already disordered eating into a return to full-blown bulimia. Which I've battled the last seven years.

I felt I was in control. Until I wasn't.

As my life fell apart, I had to finally face the reality of a long-standing, deeply embedded eating disorder.

My lap band no longer functions correctly, due to use and abuse of the band—through restricting, purging, binging, purging, binging, purging, purging and so on. Even with an empty band, I struggle to eat a balanced diet, losing a lot of the meals I eat, whether I want to or not. So, it's been determined that the only way to solve the problem is to have it removed.

It isn't urgent. I could put the surgery off for months, but I'm not into deferring stuff that needs to be done. So, the removal is scheduled for Monday and the emotional reality is starting to sink in. I'm going to be just like before—unable to control myself around food.

I feel like an abject failure.

All my life, I fail to eat in any way that could be construed as normal. And now I've failed to use the most extreme weight management tool available—surgical control of food intake.

While I've learned a ton of useful tools in the four years I've spent with my psychologist, and I had a miserable stay in the eating disorder clinic, I'm terrified of relapse. I haven't even recovered. I've made progress, but I'm still fragile. So quite frankly, knowing that once I've recovered from my surgery, I'll be able to eat with wild abandon is freaking me out. I'm starting to wonder if it's a good idea.

Everyone else thinks removing the band is a terrific idea, but all those *everyones* don't have incessant food obsessions screaming in their head day in and day out. All those *everyones* learned other ways of dealing with the normal stuff life throws around. And all those *everyones* won't have to control the movement of my fork to my mouth. Nobody can do that but me.

The reality of what I've signed myself up for has started to hit. I don't know what the future holds, but as I fear the worst, I hope for the best.

God grant me the serenity to accept the things I cannot change.

Post-surgery recovery has presented an interesting few days, and the interest is partly fuelled by regular consumption of oxycodone. Monday afternoon, I presented at the hospital for overnight admission. I wasn't thrilled but was coming to terms with it and valiantly thinking of it as a turning point in recovery. Which may well be the case. Who knows?

I lazed around, bored witless for hours awaiting my turn, and was finally wheeled to the little waiting area outside theatre. I was wearing a delightful blue and white hospital gown with its delicate ties at the back and press studs at the shoulders for easy access to every inch of my body.

Left to my own devices—no glasses to see properly and nothing to look at—instead of feeling impending doom and panic at the removal of my lap band, I was overcome with serenity and peace. (No. There were no pre-meds onboard.) Sitting in a sterile hospital bed wearing super-sexy inflatable leg things and a dainty blue and white gown, I talked to my new friend, God. I was overcome with this image of my eating disorder being surgically extracted and disposed of during the surgery. I had this overwhelming sense of a new beginning, a fresh start psychologically and physically. All the angst about the removal of the band was gone, and I just felt peaceful. And ever so tired. And bored.

Wrapped in this little spiritual glow, I was wheeled into theatre where the anaesthetist turns out to be the father of one of my former students. Moments later, I was being roused in recovery where instead of my usual rapid recovery, I struggled with pain and breathing. I was pumped full of this and that, given a nebuliser, and waited over an hour for oxygen sats to get high enough. They weren't terrible—just not good enough. I feel like I've heard that phrase my entire life.

Back on the ward, two of my four dressings start expanding and ballooning out with blood. It isn't long before they can't take the pressure and blood bursts everywhere, making a god-awful mess of my dainty gown, the pristine white sheets, and my black undies. For two hours, I have four nurses chatting with me and putting pressure on the wounds while awaiting the return of my surgeon (who is at dinner with his phone turned off enjoying a couple of wines). When he waltzes in wearing his dinner suit and a confident smile, it's all action stations—get me this needle, that local anaesthetic, these swabs, and those gloves. He cuts into my skin, swabs all the mess I've made, fishes around in the big cavity looking for the culprit, does something to it, and stitches me up with a darning needle. Then he repeats the procedure on the other side. Six sutures on the left, four on the right. For reasons I don't understand, the local anaesthetic works on the left but not the right. So that's unfun—being cut and stitched without anaesthetic. Not as bad as you'd think, but I'd choose numb if there was a next time. Apparently, I've lost about half a litre of blood. There's a big mess on the bed.

Once the bedside stitching is done, my surgeon goes home while I stand in the shower and melt away the mess. It looks like a scene from *Murder She Wrote*. When I come out feeling fresh as a daisy, my bed is pristine, and I have a lovely clean hospital gown.

Tuesday, I'm meant to go home, but by the time my surgeon does rounds, I'm having a full-blown panic attack—yesterday's peace a long lost memory. He holds my hand, asking what I want. *I don't know!* "Probably best you stay another night," he says. So, I stay another night.

Wednesday, my little pity party is all over. I know recovery is a squiggly upside down, curly wurly line that goes in many directions, so I've drawn up goals and commitments and downloaded an app or two. It would be so easy to eat myself senseless now—which is what I fear—but this is the moment to learn intuitive eating. Not binging, gorging, starving, compensating, purging, restricting, calorie-counting, judging, and all the things I've done before. Just eating properly and definitely no purging. Kirsten, Mick, and Sheree will do everything they can to support me—whether that's a listening ear or tough love. I'm forever in their debt.

God grant me the serenity to accept the things I cannot change.

And one of those things I cannot change is the endless leakage from two of my laparoscopic incisions. So much for in-one-day-and-out-the-next surgery. I'm so freaking tired.

Condensed sequence of events.

01 April 2019

- Laparoscopic removal of gastric lap band
- Postoperative bleeding from two incision sites
- Chat to four friendly nurses as they apply pressure and watch growing pools of blood on my bed (who's looking after the rest of the patients?)
- Wait two hours for surgeon to return from dinner
- Have stitches put in at bedside without anaesthetic
- Watch with macabre fascination as he digs deep into my insides stitching stuff up
- Lose half a litre of blood

02 April

- For the first time in seven years, eat without restriction
- Panic at this new realisation
- Cry all day

03 April

- Go home
- Realise I have more pain than all my other surgical procedures
- Have large quantities of opiates in my possession: temptation
- Start to notice rash and itching from dressings
- Stock up on antihistamines

04–08 April

- Sleep twenty-three hours a day
- Fail to remember much
- Kaleidoscope of blue, purple, green, yellow bruising awash my belly, back and front and bottom
- Morbidly watch as bruising heads south and threatens to crawl up my vagina
- Wonder how big haematomas can grow under stitches
- Drink whole bottle of liquid ferritin to boost flailing iron levels
- Allergic reaction to ferritin counteracts constipating effects of opiates
- Standing up causes low blood pressure: go back to bed

09 April

- Leave house for the first time
- Spend the day with Sheree completely forgetting I have a DBT class to attend and feel guilt for a week
- Spend two days in bed recovering from visiting Sheree

12 April

- Follow up surgeon visit
- Have stitches removed
- Attempted aspiration of grapefruit-sized haematoma doesn't work
- Cuts stitches open and sprays blood everywhere
- Drains haematomas
- Applies steristrips
- Ninety minutes later, steristrips are swimming in pools of blood
- Attend emergency department to have stitches put back in

13–15 April

- Dressings continue to swim in fluids
- Realise smaller wound is infected
- Lie in sun without dressings for several hours hoping to kill infection with sunlight
- Attend first gym session in a month—cannot get into plank position for first time in my life
- Feel sorry for myself

16 April

- Visit GP and ask for assessment
- Larger stitched wound deemed fine—no dressings required
- Smaller steristrip wound looking better
- Steristrips deemed pointless—dressings still required
- Continue large doses of antihistamines to relieve rashes from dressings
- Increasing panic at realisation of ease of eating
- Gain a thousand kilos
- Attend gym
- Start bleeding from large, stitched wound again
- Feel sorry for myself again
- God grant me the serenity to accept the things I cannot change.

18 April

- Hope God is listening
- Thank God for antihistamines
- Wonder if this absurd saga will ever end
- Cry for days after final appointment with my retiring psychologist
- Hope tomorrow is a better day

Five months later

- Fully healed from stitches saga
- Emotionally scarred from lap band removal
- Transitioned to new but equally lovely psychologist

FOOD RULE 6,765

Forgive relapses.

THE WILL TO LIVE

Some days, I want to live. Some days, I want to die. I'm not suicidal—not anymore. Or not at the moment, at any rate. If I'm careful with self-care and practise what has been preached the past twelve months, I can expect to die from natural causes in the distant future and not at my own hands.

This doesn't stop ideation appearing at unexpected moments. I wonder if it's always been there? I think it has. I just didn't recognise it. Since going through a period of making concrete plans, I notice those suicidal thoughts, out of place like an autumn leaf drifting through the winter snow. When they strike, I find myself having to distinguish between the fantasy dream of *wouldn't it be lovely?!* and the genuine desire for *I can't do this anymore*.

It's an odd thing, and if you've never wished to close your eyes and slip forever into a blessed and eternal sleep, then perhaps it is difficult to understand.

Suicidal plans must be bred out of depression; surely happy people don't want to die? But suicidal ideation—the thoughts that flit through your head when you least expect it—can come at any time.

One day, it might just be exhaustion. Not enough sleep the night before or a long day at work, then while driving home, chaotic thoughts are calmed by contemplating the how, why, when, what, and where of all the different lethal options there are.

Another day—when everything that can go wrong does go wrong—the thought of never having to go through another day of shit is heavenly. No plans in place. Just a blissful, mesmerising moment, realising the finality of death would bring an end to all of life's painful moments.

The most disconcerting suicidal thoughts come out of the blue—when there's no exhaustion, no sadness, no stress—just a contented day with hope and dreams for the future, and yet the mind drifts again to the pleasant nostalgia of going to sleep and never waking up. Of never having to deal with life again—the good, the bad, the ugly. The mundane, the exciting, the horrific. All the things that life is—gone.

Nostalgic, dreamy moments are not the same as being suicidal. Not at all. I've been there, and there's no comparison.

Being suicidal is an intense darkness in the deepest part of your spirit and soul. Born out of a deep depression that lasts long enough to leave nothing but numbing blackness and strips away all hope there is any chance of reprieve. Life isn't worth living, depression tells you.

Day after endless day, it relentlessly marches on, and each relentless day is harder to survive than the one before. Suicidal plans are made. The suicidal dream is becoming a reality. An increasingly tempting possibility and the how, why, when, what, and where are constructed and put into place. Each day is a trial and survived only by setting small goals and having enough loving family and support around that the final decision is never reached.

With support and time, the unrelenting desire for eternal rest diminishes. Will it ever go entirely? I suspect not. I have become sensitised to every suicidal thought that passes through my consciousness. But ideation doesn't involve plans. Ideation doesn't bring with it spiralling depression and obsessive thought patterns. Ideation doesn't mean the end of all that is near and dear. It's simply dreaming of a fantasy that will never be pursued. It's not reality. It's not fact. It's not healthy. It's just a dream. A tangled web of desires. A dark dream that can hit at any time. A dark dream banished by focusing on the light. And every single day holds both light and dark.

Today, I awoke to the sight of Coco, my cat's, brown furry ears resting on my pillow, peering out the window at the rising sun and the clear blue autumn skies. The day held so much hope.

Hope can be deceiving.

It matters not how, or why, I ended up in a cycle of soul-destroying binging and purging; the reasons are much the same as all the others, that I lack the emotional skills to deal with life. What matters is what I do now, because that determines how genuine my desire for recovery is.

My first action was to reach out to a community who understand binge eating and bulimia. I was reminded of a guided visualisation for self-compassion. It was exactly what I needed. I've listened twice and it brought up a lot of thoughts, grief, and ancient history. It left me with powerful memories—memories so clear I could almost reach out and touch them. So real I'm still processing and grieving.

Immediately post-binge, my thoughts turn inward, becoming hateful and spiteful. They speak to me in a manner I'd never contemplate speaking to anybody else. The hypercritical voice speaks in a degrading and humiliating tone. It reminds me I'm a failure and a moron. It says I'm not good enough and my intrinsic value is in superficial appearances. It believes I'll never get off this roller-coaster; I'm here to stay. I'm beyond redemption.

That voice is my protector, and it's afraid. It's terrified I'll get fat, so it motivates me to keep doing what I'm doing. It's afraid I'll never recover, so it discourages me from going through the heartache of trying. That voice has always loved me but never helped me. It's never served me but has always meant well.

That voice is my mother.

I can see and hear her as if she were standing in front of me. With loving concern, she says I need to lose weight; *if you could just lose a few pounds, dear, you'd start to look quite attractive.* She means well. I know she does. She always did. She worries I'm not slim enough or attractive enough to be happy in life because that's what she learned.

But today, I said goodbye. I thanked her and watched her walk away.

I love and miss her, but I'll never see her again. I don't need her voice or concern; I never did. It hasn't helped me one little bit. My mother is long gone, but I've been seeking the love and approval I so desperately wanted from her all my life. I'll never receive it. Today, I said goodbye and embraced that truth.

Many deeply held beliefs about myself come from my mother and grandmother, and those beliefs have to go; they're intolerably painful and destructive. They may have been intended as a means of protecting me from all sorts of perceived pain, but the intention was misguided, and the harm was incalculable. Now the time is right, so I conjure a vivid image of my mother in her forties—a time when I was in my teens and most damaged by her words—and thank her for her efforts and ask her to stop. Her words can impact me no more. I let her go. Let her voice, fears, and concerns vacate my head. I watch her turn around and walk away, wearing her white button-up shirt and knee-length blue skirt. She's slim and beautiful and in the prime of her life. She's healthy and vital, full of hope and love. She's gone.

I've always had a timid voice of reason quietly arguing in the background. Today, I welcomed that voice and gave it a face. That face is five-year-old me. A little girl with golden-red curls, a fierce independence, and a fire in her belly. No dream impossible, no fate improbable, no problem insurmountable.

Life stretched out with infinite opportunities, days and nights secure in the knowledge that anything can happen. A little girl craving love and attention. Desperate to be good—to be noticed, wanted, and nurtured. Starved of affection that little girl is the only one that knows how to heal me. She can hand out the hugs so desperately wanted, knowing what's needed. Knowing how to forgive and move on. She's a messy concoction of nature and nurture, with a propensity for depression and high anxiety—seeking perfection and independence almost as badly as she yearns for acceptance and unconditional love. Acutely sensitive to sights, sounds, and smells, and intuitively empathic in a world she's too young to understand.

So, I take her hand, and she looks up with unbroken trust and a ready smile. *Shall we go?* We walk together. Past years of judgment about appearance and body function. Past endless criticisms of every task ever attempted or completed. Away from the incessant catalogue of imperfections, mistakes, poor choices, and constant disappointments. And a legacy resulting in a dearth of self-care, self-confidence, self-esteem, and self-awareness.

I take her by the hand. The little girl with the freckles dusting her fair skin and her perfectly straight teeth with the small gap in front. Her unruly curly hair, straightened with a part in the centre and pigtails neatly behind her ears. Green eyes bright with hope and a willing smile ready to charm and cajole for her deepest desires.

Today, I farewelled my mother—ten years after she died. More than fifty years after she instilled the critical voice of judgment in my heart. Today, I welcomed the little girl who waited all these years for the love she was always worthy of—simply because she exists.

Today, I grieved. Tomorrow, I start to become whole.

COMING HOME

If you'd told me in 2015 that my poor, long-suffering psychologist would still be listening to my woes after four years, I would have said *no way!* (possibly in much stronger language).

It seems this recovery gig is far more complex than anticipated. When first I sat upon that lovely soft couch, I shared a couple of issues, strategies were discussed, then I went away and practised. I'm usually very obedient. Next time I visited, I divulged a little more, and it seemed my problems were perhaps bigger than anticipated. New strategies to try. As my trust solidified, she started to delve a lot deeper and unearthed problems even bigger and more deep-rooted than first thought. It took perhaps half a dozen appointments to dig down into the nitty-gritty of my shitty stuff, and as it turns out, those first few strategies couldn't hack the pace. Tougher stuff was needed, so she wheeled out the big guns.

Part of the recovery process is self-compassion, self-acceptance, self-love. These are the most difficult—probably crucial—parts of the journey for me. Compassion needs to extend to every part of me, inside and out.

Letting go of a deeply held belief or feeling is not a conscious choice. It may be something you've always known you must do, but the time has to be right. Then one day, just like holding tight onto a big red balloon, you discover you can open your hand and let that string go, watching the balloon float off into the distance. So, I did. I think I did? The tricky thing about metaphorical strings is you can't be sure they're gone.

Sadness with no outlet gnaws a pit in your soul and gradually leaches into every aspect of your being. Anxiety second-guesses every decision and erodes any sense of self or confidence that once burned brightly. And together they quench that fire in the belly and steal the hopes and dreams of a life with infinite possibilities.

I've had an eating disorder all my years—in one form or another. I'm working through recovery, and while I still have a way to go, I'm much further along than I was. Each time I relapse, then crawl back out I ask, *why? What the fuck was I thinking?* And then it occurs to me, I keep looking for the confident girl who taught and performed, looked after everyone, and buzzed around sky-high on energy all day long. The girl who quite literally eats every emotion that touches her spirit and refuses to acknowledge life is anything but a gift she has no right to frown upon. There's no room for sadness.

Depression and anxiety are nasty sounding things other people experience. Not me. I'm the optimist always looking on the bright side. Filled with energy and joy, because everyone prefers happy people. *You have a beautiful smile, Simone!* I was calm under pressure. I knew how to deal with life and stress.

Except I didn't. I was forty-nine years old before I associated either of those words with myself.

Decades of maladaptive coping mechanisms crashed down around my ears and the words *severe depression* and *chronic anxiety* were bandied about, in relation to me. I was in the depths of self-induced starvation, self-harming, highly suicidal, too depressed to function, and suffering the physical misery of high anxiety, a pounding heart, shaking hands, internal catastrophising, panic attacks. I was one of those people.

Now I have labels and tools, but I keep searching for that confident girl. The one with the boundless energy who smiles for everyone, always says yes, and never protects herself. I make progress in recovery and keep wondering when she'll reappear—full of hopes and dreams and positivity. Desperate to live a life of purpose, to leave a lasting legacy.

But she's gone and isn't coming back. She can't. Her strength was a façade. A false belief that other people's perceptions were more important than reality. A desperate desire to please, by expending energy on other people and never taking a moment to look inward and see the festering mass of unacknowledged fear. Seeking that woman holds me back.

The new Simone can embrace the golden-haired child that was and the grey-haired woman yet to come. I don't know what the new girl looks like. Or how she dreams and reacts to life. I'm just discovering her— helping her find a voice and teaching her to be brave enough to use it. Reimagining lost hopes and dreams of youth, fine-tuning them with the hard-earned wisdom of age and experience.

The new girl has shadows of the old but is fortified with newfound knowledge and a refusal to submit to the lure of the dark side. I'm going to miss that old girl; she was so full of spirit and hope. But she was also a lie. The new girl's saggier, wrinklier, and most days, a whole lot more miserable. But she's honest and vulnerable and has the power to acknowledge and accept realities of the inevitable stresses of this thing we call life. A life packed full of highs and lows.

Today, I cried. I cried because I could feel the hard, solid, shell I spent decades plastering around every inch of me cracking, leaving me soft and vulnerable and revealing a very broken pair of wings.

The past week, my anxiety levels sky-rocketed, and as my anxiety went up, my eating went down. I need recovery. I need it with every ounce of my being—physically, mentally, psychologically, spiritually. My eating disorder weighs me down and impacts every aspect of my life. I can't bear it. And I can't bear to let it go.

Sometimes I feel the eating disorder is a solid, tangible, physical, separate part of me, and when I come across another piece of the recovery puzzle—something I believe is actually going to progress me a little further away from illness and propel me closer to wellness—it panics. It flexes its muscles and says, *Look at me! I'm stronger than you! I'm not leaving!*

After years of therapy, I feel my eating disorder panicking and reminding me, if it goes, there's nothing left to protect me. I've learned no other way to cope with life, and I rarely cope well. I shed tears of grief for behaviours I've clung to like a drowning woman all my life. I sob in fear of the emotions and angst that will come flooding in when the cracks are wide and my protection is gone.

When life gets out of control, I morph into diminishing self-care— self-sabotage, if you will. I forget my medications, get manic doing everything for everyone else, stop doing housework, stop writing, and stop personal care. It's embarrassing; nobody wants to admit they no longer bother to remove makeup or brush their teeth before crawling into bed. It grosses me out. I do it anyway. It's a pretty clear indicator I'm not in tip-top shape at this point. Recovery is teaching me to recognise symptoms before my teeth start suffering.

I have no idea what recovered looks and feels like. And I certainly have no idea what will replace disordered eating, self-harm, and my collection of new behaviours to allow me to cope with the inevitable stresses that will darken my days. But as the rest of my protective shell is ripped away, I want to unfurl those broken wings and give them a test run to see where they take me. I want those wings to take me home.

I've known a lot of homes. An endless cascade of houses where I lay my head and unpacked my bags. A dozen educational institutions where a seat was mine and mine alone, and I found a place to feel belonging and purpose. Friends where no amount of time and distance separates us, and despite the years between, a phone call picks up where the last one left off. And I've found home in my husband and children. When all my world crumbled, grief stumbled in, or joy and excitement were too big to contain, they've been the place that holds me.

There's one more home to find. Myself.

If home is a place of safety, security, and familiarity, then that's the place I seek. A place deep inside my belly, with an eternal knowing that no matter the tsunami of life eddying around me, there's security in my being.

Coming home means an end to numbing. An end to punishment and self-recrimination. The beginning of acceptance and love. A willingness to embody the body I was born with and appreciate its ability to carry me with ease and grace. Resisting illness. Growing and nourishing children. Carrying me into the ecstasy of carnal love and allowing me to experience the agony of brokenness and the relief when agony abates.

Coming home is an acknowledgement of all my faults and flaws in equal measure with all my gifts and talents. Accepting the whole of my unique self as no better and no worse than any other.

Coming home means a deep sense of peace. A peace I barely know or recognise but have in brief moments of time felt nestled in my soul. A peace I yearn to know more deeply, more easily, more frequently. A sense of comfort with myself—the wrinkles, the scars. My intellect and creativity. My empathy and caring. My inclination to rush and catastrophise. The well-intentioned need to solve everyone's problems. My gift of teaching and music and writing. The whole of me. The me my friends choose to spend time with, decade after decade. The me my husband adores. The me my children love. The me my father is proud of.

Forgiveness is an act of courage and strength. To come home to myself requires forgiveness for all I am not. All I have lost. All I regret.

Appreciation is an act of love and kindness. To come home to myself requires appreciation for all that I am. All I have been. All I have achieved.

Self-love is an act of compassion and acceptance. To come home to myself requires self-love from my chipped painted toenails to the roots of my greying hairline.

I choose to come home. To take the hand of the little girl who was never good enough in her mother's eyes and say, *You are enough. Right now. As is.* To squish her to my breast and meld her to my heart. Complete healing. That is to come home to me.

FOOD RULE 10,946

Eat intuitively.

EPILOGUE

THE DECLARATION OF FREEDOM

I live in a house surrounded by nature. I sit in bed of a morning watching wattlebirds singing in the trees outside my bedroom window. I can see the water. I can hear the waves. I can watch the sunrise. These things are always here. They always have been. I've lived in this house for twenty years.

In a world free from food obsession, the birdsong brings me peace. The sunrise heralds a new dawn—a new day with fresh beginnings and all the possibilities every new day brings. There are no rainbows and unicorns. This is the real world. It isn't sprinkled with magic wands, fairy wings, and pixie dust. It's filled with fortune and favour, trials and tribulations, love and loss. My world is filled with all the things that are.

In my freedom, I soak up love and energy, gifts and privilege, when they are sent my way. I appreciate the joy of family dinner nights, the peace of stargazing on a camping trip, and the contentment of good company. My spirit is filled. My soul rested. I practice acceptance of what is and courage for what could be. I have serenity, for that is the reward of acceptance and courage.

In my freedom, I have the strength to conquer the trials I inevitably face. I accept what cannot be changed. I grieve for that which is gone. I cry with sadness and give voice to frustrations, because I'm human. I belong to humanity, and we all have the capacity and need to explore the full range of human emotions. I have the right to express emotions. All pain is dealt with; how productively it's dealt with is a choice I must make.

In a world free from food obsession, where my personal worth is founded in my actions and beliefs and not in my physical appearance, I focus entirely on being the best person I can be. I explore my talents without fear of judgment—internally or externally. I try my hardest and know it's enough. In a world free from negative body image, I am enough. I am enough as is. Not in a day or a week or a year. Not in a number on a scale or a dress size. *I. Am. Enough.*

In this free world, I share love and gratitude openly in my relationships—my close personal relationships and my collegial working relationships. I give vent to frustrations, concerns, and upsets, without fear of retribution. I am whole. I give and I can take. I care for others and show the depths of kindness, care, and empathy I have always given. But also freely acknowledge my limits and accept the gifts of kindness, care, and empathy when they are proffered.

In this free world, I exercise because I love how it makes my body feel—strong, powerful, alive, and cared for. I eat because food nourishes every ounce of my being. I eat because food brings people together, and a shared meal is shared love. I'm free from incessant food thoughts, and instead fill my mind with the wonders of the world in which I live—the people, the places, and the passions I love. I'm free from the necessity to eat for punishment, shame, or to numb myself.

Observation replaces punishment. I see what happened, take a deep breath, learn, move on.

Self-compassion replaces shame. I treat myself with the care and love I would anyone else. It's not selfish or narcissistic. It's necessary. If it's necessary for everyone else, I'm no exception. I'm not special. I'm normal. I need self-compassion; it is the antidote to shame.

Acceptance replaces numbing. I sit with emotions, and they don't kill me. It's uncomfortable, and that's okay. In a three-dimensional world, I can experience all sides of the emotional coin. This too shall pass.

This world of freedom is not glowing angelically. It's filled with all the darkness and light that my world, and everyone else's world, is filled with. But with my spirit freed from the hard shell it's encased in, the soft glow from my freshly unfurled wings lights the way on the darkest of days.

This is how freedom will look for me.

ACKNOWLEDGMENTS

My life, like so many, has been filled with labour and love, and so here, I would like to express my undying thanks to those who have supported this particular labour of love. For my book would not exist without their patience and care.

To the man who loves me no matter what, holds me when I fall, then lifts me back up again. Mick, I couldn't do my life without you, and sharing my story would certainly not have come to pass. All those years ago, you found a little writing challenge group on Facebook for me to join and encouraged me to push a little into an awkward space just to see what might happen. And look what happened—I wrote a book! A cathartic healing you have helped me bring into the world. Thank you for our decades together and may we have many more to come.

To my three and a half children—Jamie, Conor, Liam, and Hamish. Thank you for the opportunity to be a part of your lives and to show me the meaning of irrepressibly unconditional love. I am grateful that you can love me through my ugliest moments. May we share many more family dinners filled with robust conversations on renewable energies, differential equations, and helicopters on Mars.

To Kiki, for being a part of the next chapter of my story, sharing a life-altering bubble of happiness with me, and loving me when I needed it the most. You are my kindred spirit. You are, and always will be, just like a daughter to me.

To my immediate family—June, Gordon, Carrol, Christian, Kristin, and Vanessa. You shaped the person I am today, and no matter what, I am always grateful for our love and connections. I miss you, one and all, every day.

To my irreplaceable group of friends who stand by me through thick and thin, in every sense of the word. Kerry, Kirsten, Karen, Bronwyn, Vanessa, Emma, Sheree, Maree, Amanda, Tania, Zoe, Mel, you have taught me I am loved for who I am from the inside out. We have grown together, and I am intensely grateful to know you. May we share many more walks in nature with gin and tonics under the stars.

To my musical colleagues and flocks of flute students—thank you. What wonderful people you are. Thank you for the opportunity to let me be me and to explore all my talents, such as they are. Thank you for letting me become just a little part of your story.

To my writing mentor, Joanne Fedler, for teaching me the seven C's and the craft of writing. And to my manuscript assessor, Julie Gray, for believing in me and this adventure. And to all my fellow writers in the Author Awakening Adventure. Sharing your stories and listening to mine without judgment has helped me in more ways than you will ever understand. I am so grateful to you.

To the wonderful publishing team at Koehler Books, thank you for turning my dream into a reality. The gentle guidance, meticulous editing, stunning graphic design and faith in my writing mean the world to me.

Thank you to all those who supported me in launching my book campaign, and most especially Michelle Warren, for her huge contribution and belief in me. There is no sentiment more apt than thank you. You are a rock star.

And finally, thank you to Lindsay for the use of your cottage on Bruny Island. Many cathartic stories were typed up in the little bay window looking out over the D'Entrecasteaux Channel while the echidna nibbled ants on the back step. All those peaceful, quiet writing breaks helped me bring my story to fruition. What a piece of paradise.

CPSIA information can be obtained
at www.ICGtesting.com
Printed in the USA
BVHW071345030122
625349BV00008B/205